fashionable clothing
from the sears catalogs

Tina Skinner & Lindy McCord

LATE 1940s

with price guide

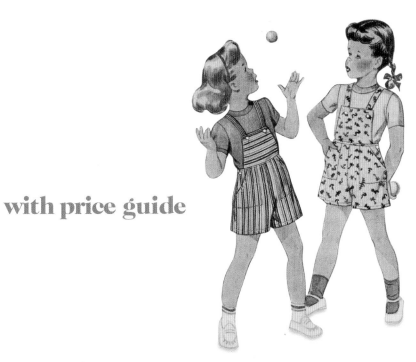

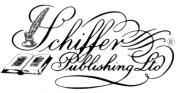

Schiffer Publishing Ltd

4880 Lower Valley Road, Atglen, PA 19310 USA

Library of Congress Cataloging-in-Publication Data

Skinner, Tina.
Fashionable clothing from the Sears catalogs: late 1940's/Tina Skinner & Lindy McCord; photography by Tammy Ward and Lindy McCord.
p. cm.
ISBN 0-7643-1955-8 (pbk.)
1. Clothing and dress--Catalogs. 2. Costume--Collectors and collecting--United States--History-20th century--Catalogs. 3. Sears, Roebuck and Company--Catalogs. 4. Large type books. I. McCord, Lindy. II. Title.
TT555.S557 2004
391'.009'044--dc22
2003018695

Edited by Melissa Cardona
Designed by Bonnie M. Hensley
Cover design by Bruce Waters
Type set in Coventry Garden/Aldine 721 Lt BT

ISBN: 0-7643-1955-8
Printed in China
1 2 3 4

Fall/Winter 1946-1947: 3, 8, 9, 13, 15, 16, 21, 24, 25, 27, 29, 30, 37, 39, 43, 44, 46, 49, 53, 55, 58, 59, 63, 71, 73, 77, 81, 126, 127, 129, 132, 133, 147, 149, 150, 151, 152, 153, 154, 159, 163, 165, 167, 170, 172, 173, 175, 176, 178, 181, 187, 188, 190, 191, 205, 221, 223, 225, 241, 243, 259, 260, 261, 268, 269, 272, 273, 279, 282, 283, 296, 302, 306, 390, 392, 393, 394, 402, 403, 407, 459, 473, 477, 482, 485, 490, 491, 493, 495, 505, 508, 509, 515, 520, 521, 524, 531, 539, 541, 543, 561, 562, 580, 581

Spring/Summer 1947: 37, 39, 40, 42, 44, 49, 53, 57, 60, 62, 65, 67, 70, 71, 78, 83, 84, 85, 87, 90, 96, 101,102, 103, 108, 113, 115, 117, 120, 123, 127, 133, 134, 136, 161, 163, 165, 169, 179, 188, 189, 193, 193D, 198, 204, 205, 206, 207, 218, 224, 226, 243, 289, 291, 293, 300, 304, 309, 310, 316, 322, 325B, 328, 336, 337, 352, 355, 361B, 361C, 362, 363, 367, 368, 370-372, 375, 376, 377, 379, 386, 395, 396, 401, 404, 408, 413, 414, 415, 427, 433, 437

Fall/Winter 1948: 2, 7, 8, 9, 12, 17, 21, 23, 31, 63, 71, 73, 74, 91, 98,101, 103, 109, 112, 113, 121, 123, 125, 157B, 160, 163, 177, 182, 183, 185, 187, 199, 217, 221, 225, 227, 235, 237, 245, 257, 263, 287, 289, 295, 297B, 298, 301, 305, 306, 309A, 313, 316, 328, 341, 357, 360, 370, 378, 381, 401, 404, 417, 419, 453, 455, 471, 475, 494, 496, 501, 505, 507, 511, 515, 516, 519, 250, 521, 543, 554, 557, 564, 566, 573

Spring/Summer 1949: 20, 21, 30, 84, 85, 97, 119, 125, 131, 133, 143, 150, 154, 157, 164, 170, 171, 187, 190, 191, 195, 201, 213, 219, 220, 223, 225, 233, 234, 251, 256, 260, 261, 275, 299, 301, 302, 304, 333, 338

Published by Schiffer Publishing Ltd.
4880 Lower Valley Road
Atglen, PA 19310
Phone: (610) 593-1777; Fax: (610) 593-2002
E-mail: Info@schifferbooks.com
Please visit our web site catalog at **www.schifferbooks.com**
We are always looking for people to write books on new and related subjects. If you have an idea for a book, please contact us at the above address.

This book may be purchased from the publisher.
Include $3.95 for shipping.
Please try your bookstore first.
You may write for a free catalog.

In Europe, Schiffer books are distributed by
Bushwood Books
6 Marksbury Avenue
Kew Gardens
Surrey TW9 4JF England
Phone: 44 (0) 20 8392 8585
Fax: 44 (0) 20 8392 9876
E-mail: Bushwd@aol.com
Free postage in the UK. Europe: air mail at cost.

CONTENTS

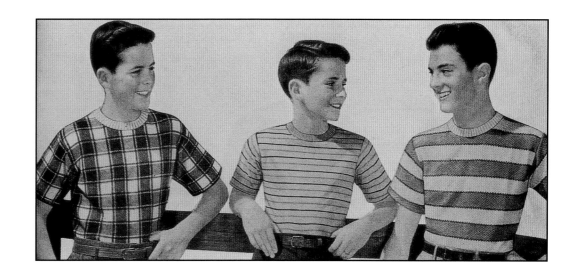

Post-war America brought about significant changes in fashion trends as the economy boomed. Men returned from the war, ready to reclaim the jobs that women had so diligently taken over. The icon "Rosie the Riveter" still held value for women, but many women – who'd enthusiastically welcomed the men back – were back in the home, becoming mothers and enjoying the proliferation of modern conveniences such as electric refrigerators, Tupperware, and aluminum foil.

Politically, the American government was most concerned about containment of the Soviet Union. Rationing slowly came to an end and materials that were either too expensive or too scarce during the war were once again readily available. Sanforized work and play clothing was still prominent, and full-blended wool garments made a comeback as prices dropped.

One of the most important developments in fashion in the late 1940s was the introduction of 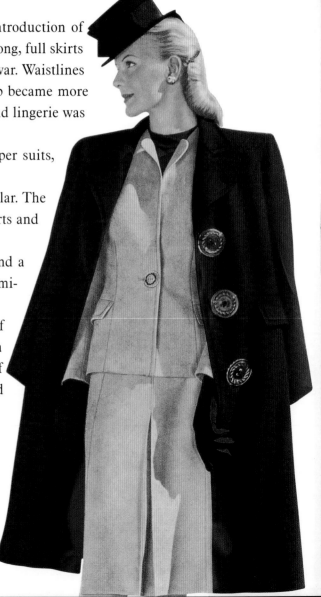 Christian Dior's "New Look." This style allowed women to show off their curves, with long, full skirts wrapping women in yards of feminine fabrics that had all but disappeared during the war. Waistlines were cinched, flat-soled shoes were abandoned for more exciting pumps, and make-up became more socially acceptable. Celebrities like Rita Hayworth made sweaters more fashionable, and lingerie was starting to enhance and not just support.

Men's fashions remained similar to those from years past, with lots of crisp dapper suits, colorful warm sweaters, or attractive pullovers for the less formal hours.

For the teenagers of post-war America, T-shirts and jeans became exceedingly popular. The term "bobby-soxers" was born, bringing to mind styles characterized by large flare skirts and big motifs. Teen girls' fashions allowed girls to express themselves as individuals.

Children's fashion changed as well, with knickers becoming a relic of the past, and a more casual style emerging. Colors bloomed and lively prints became more and more prominent.

All in all, the country was moving forward with a positive attitude. Even with a lot of lives left to rebuild, and a long way to go before truly attaining economic stability, America was a nation reborn. Quite literally, the advent of the baby boom and subsequent burst of children's fashions in the catalogs of the time is testament to the growing population in need of togs.

The following images offer a historic overview of everyday fashions in America. The original catalog language has been abridged in the image captions, along with the original prices. For those who seek out the vintage articles today, a suggested value range is provided in brackets. These values are meant only as a guideline, and the true value of an item should be gauged by its condition, along with the interest and demand for the item in the current fashion world.

Dress Up/Career

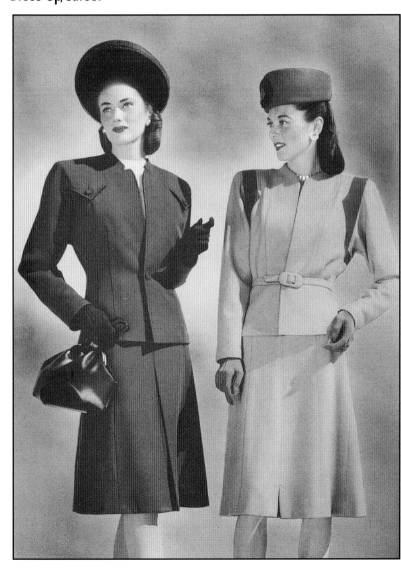

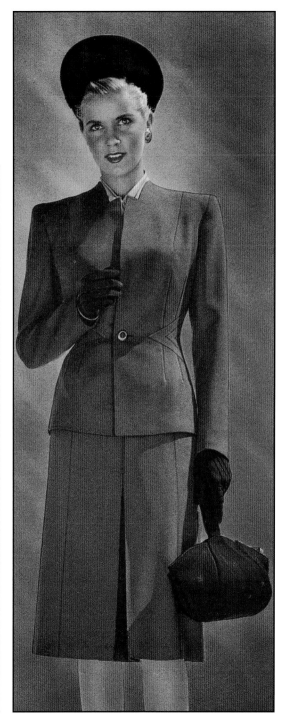

Diagonal-weave wool, far-reaching sleeves, shoulders accented with contrasting colored inserts. Beige with brown, medium brown with beige, or black with rosy red inserts. $25. Wool crepe, rich-textured and dressy, the ideal fabric for the suit. Gored skirt with neat front pleat. $27. [$10-20] *Fall/winter 1946-1947*

Silky, fine-grained, all wool gabardine suit. Sleek, stitched waistline. Medium green, medium blue, or medium brown. $30. [$10-20] *Fall/winter 1946-1947*

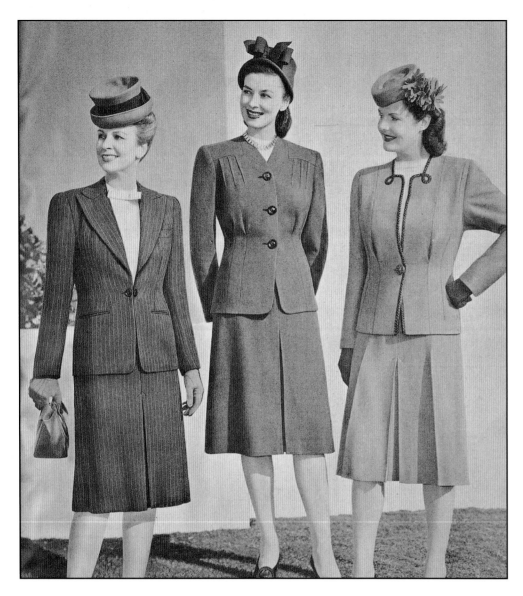

Glittering nailheads cascade down the front of this classic two-piece all wool crepe dress, in gold, light coral red, or medium blue. Expensive-looking dressmaker pin-tucks front and back, and tricolor suede belt give a new, feminine look. Light gray, medium blue, or gold. $13-15. [$15-20] *Fall/winter 1946-1947*

Suits from Kerrybrooke Fashions. Link-button suit, strictly tailored, faint white hairline stripe worked in slimming lines. Navy blue or black. $19. Young cardigan suit, smartly collarless, tucks its waist for sleekness. Black, navy blue, or royal blue. $17. All wool crepe dressy suit with rayon-lined jacket outlined in rich rayon braid. Black, medium green, medium brown, or navy blue, $27. [$10-20] *Fall/winter 1946-1947*

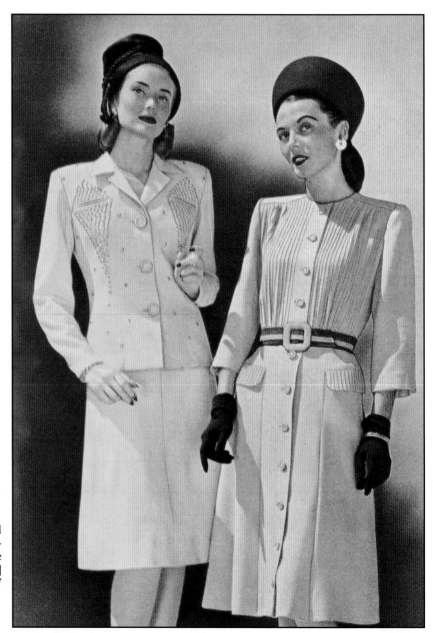

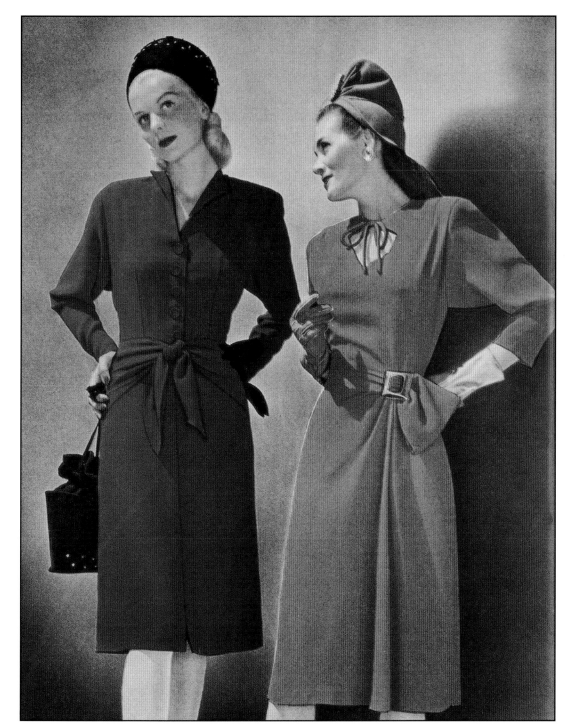

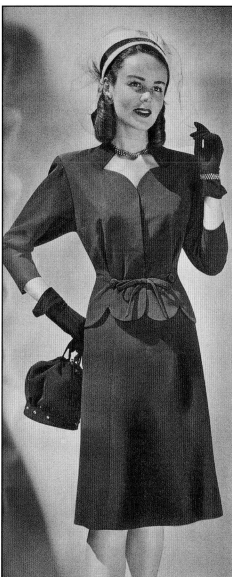

Two-piece gains fresh importance with inspired dressmaker styling. Sweetheart neckline can be changed with frothy lingerie or imaginative jewelry. Smartly scalloped front finished with a self tie, in black and dark brown. $9. [$5-10] *Fall/winter 1946-1947*

Dresses with soft draping capture the wonderful new feeling in fashion, all by Kerrybrooke. Draped peplum is a fashion headliner, especially when it wraps and ties like this one. Mallinson's Whirlaway, rich-textured rayon crepe. Black or royal blue. Dramatic side swept skirt is caught in a buckle and falls in soft folds. Flattering keyhole neckline and deep shoulder flange. Cherry rose or black. Both, $9. [$5-10] *Fall/winter 1946-1947*

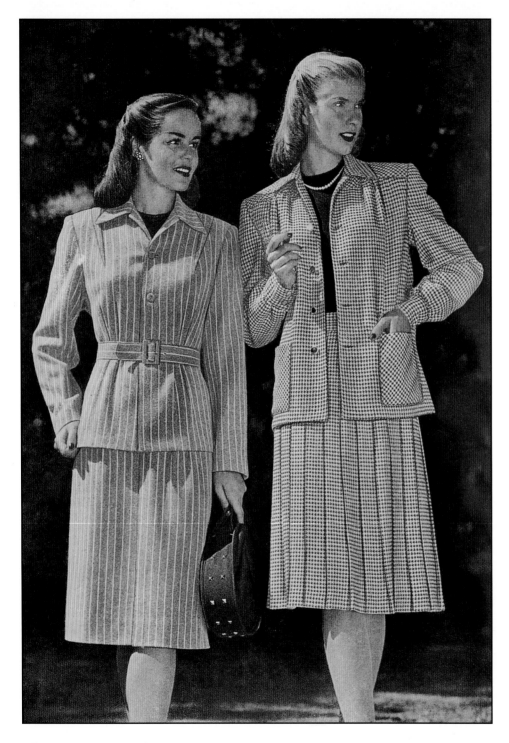

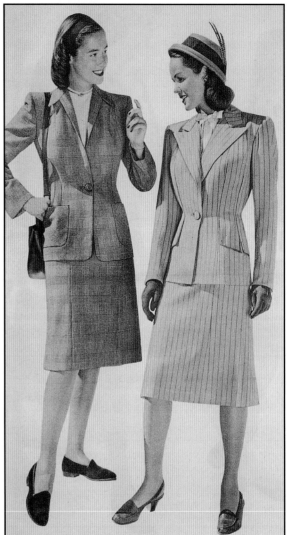

Belted or buttoned…patterned, braided, or sparkle-struck…the pick of the season's prized suits are here. Glen plaid, rich-woven 100% pure wool, deep-diving collar, one-button closing. Gray, red, and black plaid, or blue, gray, and black plaid. Menswear stripes, splendid blend of 40% pure wool worsted and 60% rayon. New long-lined look for jacket that flings lapels far and wide. Gray ground with black stripe, beige tan ground with brown stripe, or medium blue ground with lighter blue stripe. $30. [$10-15] *Spring/summer 1947*

Teamed up for a real career suit, smart skirts and jackets. New softened lines, belted waists, wing sleeves, and shirtmaker cuffs. Dapper checked outfit, unlined boxy jacket, pleated skirt with neat zipper placket. Black and white, or brown and white. $12. Gray with white stripes, 100% wool skirt and jacket. Belted jacket, deep-cut armholes show the smart dolman influence, in medium gray. $14. [$20-30] *Fall/winter 1946-1947*

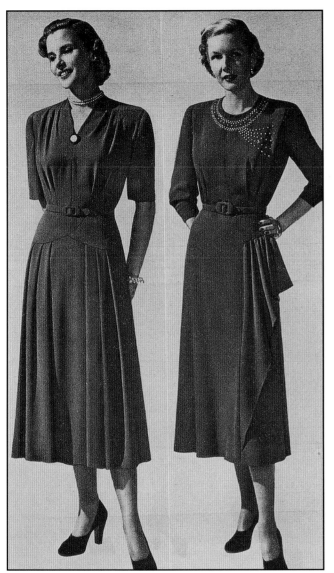

Versatile basic dress, fine rayon alpaca. Smart with your own jewelry. Black, plum wine, or deep blue. Sparkling nailheads on good, quality spun rayon. Silver-color on blue, or gold color on cocoa brown dress. New circular-cut skirt, spun rayon with colorful appliqués, youthful feel that's extremely becoming to women, slim over the hips. Medium gray, medium blue. $8. [$10-20] *Fall/winter 1947-1948*

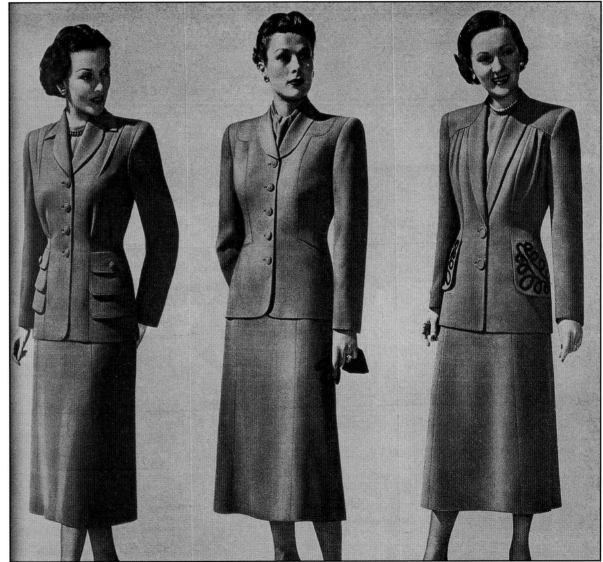

Budget-minded all wool suits…newest flattering-to-you fashions. Choose braid trimming, soft neckline, or stylish hip interest. Tiered flaps add just the right interest to the hipline. All wool crepe, figure slimming gored skirt is the new longer length. Shawl collar, tailored beautifully in firm textured all wool covert…look right for dressy occasions, yet simple enough for every day. $26.50. Collarless suit, dressed up with color-blending rayon braid hip flaps. Medium gray or medium brown. $19.50. [$20-30] *Fall/winter 1948*

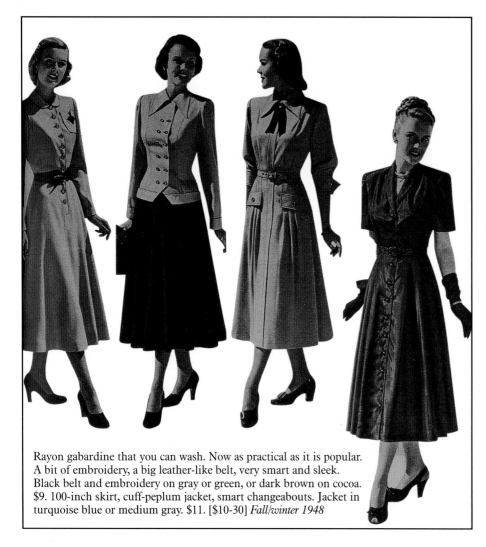

Rayon gabardine that you can wash. Now as practical as it is popular.
A bit of embroidery, a big leather-like belt, very smart and sleek.
Black belt and embroidery on gray or green, or dark brown on cocoa.
$9. 100-inch skirt, cuff-peplum jacket, smart changeabouts. Jacket in
turquoise blue or medium gray. $11. [$10-30] *Fall/winter 1948*

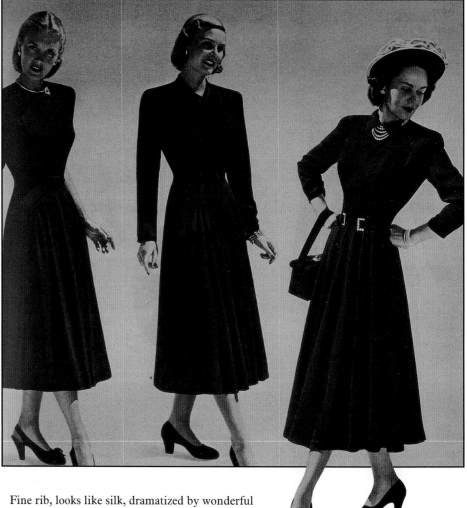

Fine rib, looks like silk, dramatized by wonderful
lines and details. Styles in the best rayon crepe or
rayon alpaca. New draped dolman sleeves with front
skirt yoke, in deep blue, black, or brown. Smart
side-button bodice, front skirt yoke with new peg
drape. Fabric belt and buttons, in black, purple
wine, or deep blue. 110-inch skirt, full all around.
Bias-cut to give you a smooth hipline, darts above
the hipline to mold your middle. Buckles sparkle
with rhinestones, in black, deep blue, or deep
brown. $11-14. [$10-30] *Fall/winter 1948*

Smart wool in a basket weave…soft, warm…Kerrybrooke quality tailoring. Button-front with convertible collar, fabric belt and buttons, multicolor embroidery. Aqua blue, coral rose, or gold. $7.25. Stars twinkle on the front bodice, all over the sleeves, and down the peplum. $8. Front yoke effect dress, inset pockets, rich wool. Brown embroidery on aqua, gold, or rose. $7.50. Easy-to-wash spun rayon, Kerrybrooke expert tailoring. A skillful contrast of print and plain to flatter your figure, in slenderizing black with white. $6. [$5-15] *Fall/winter 1948*

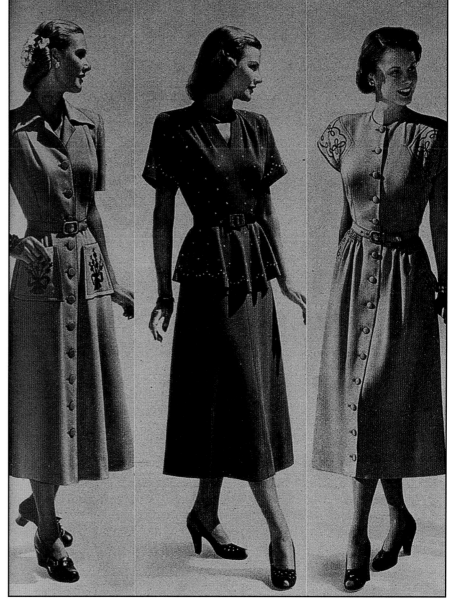

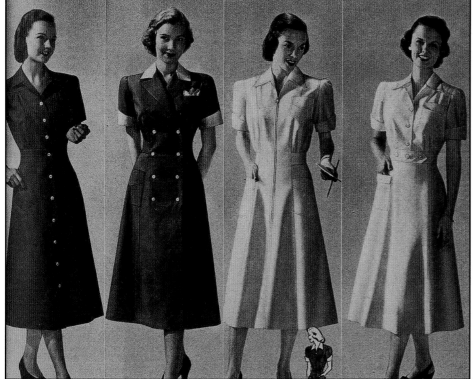

Kerrybrooke Sanforized cotton utility uniforms. For the working woman, in beauty parlors, factories, restaurants, or laboratories. All styles in blue, white, and green, available in sturdy cotton with linen-like finish or in fine broadcloth. $2-4. [$5-10] *Fall/winter 1948*

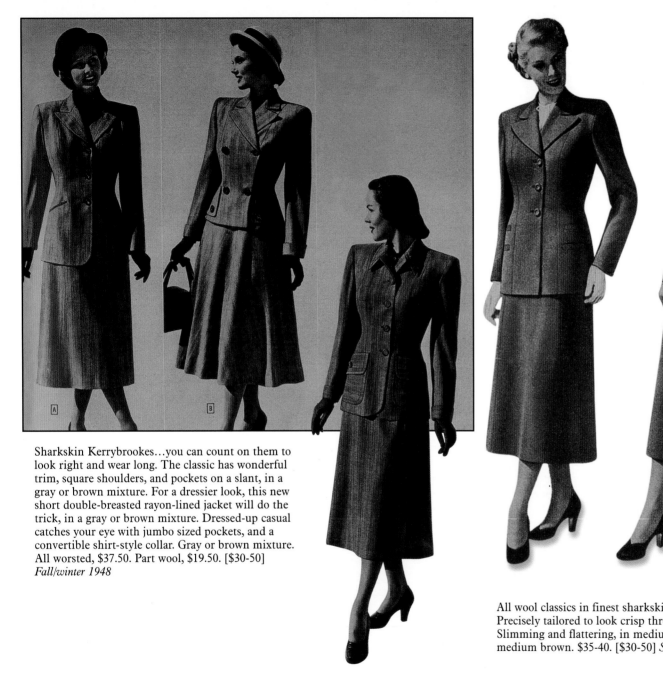

Sharkskin Kerrybrookes…you can count on them to look right and wear long. The classic has wonderful trim, square shoulders, and pockets on a slant, in a gray or brown mixture. For a dressier look, this new short double-breasted rayon-lined jacket will do the trick, in a gray or brown mixture. Dressed-up casual catches your eye with jumbo sized pockets, and a convertible shirt-style collar. Gray or brown mixture. All worsted, $37.50. Part wool, $19.50. [$30-50] *Fall/winter 1948*

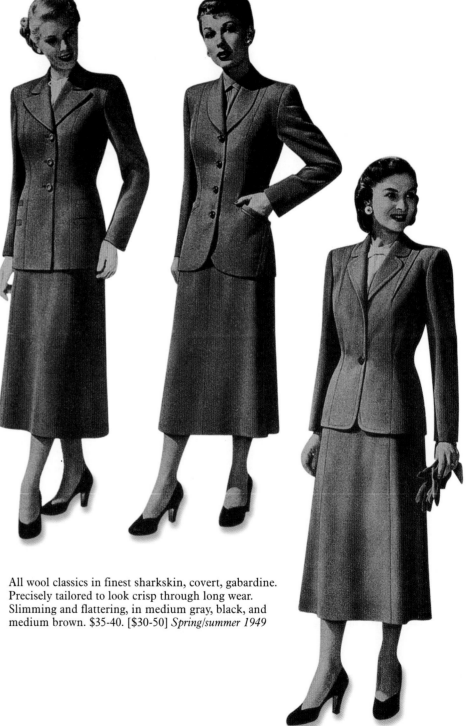

All wool classics in finest sharkskin, covert, gabardine. Precisely tailored to look crisp through long wear. Slimming and flattering, in medium gray, black, and medium brown. $35-40. [$30-50] *Spring/summer 1949*

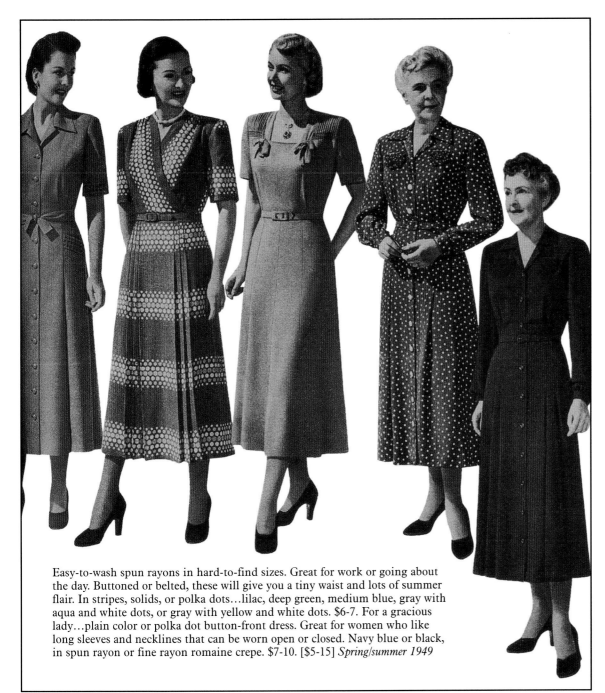

Easy-to-wash spun rayons in hard-to-find sizes. Great for work or going about the day. Buttoned or belted, these will give you a tiny waist and lots of summer flair. In stripes, solids, or polka dots…lilac, deep green, medium blue, gray with aqua and white dots, or gray with yellow and white dots. $6-7. For a gracious lady…plain color or polka dot button-front dress. Great for women who like long sleeves and necklines that can be worn open or closed. Navy blue or black, in spun rayon or fine rayon romaine crepe. $7-10. [$5-15] *Spring/summer 1949*

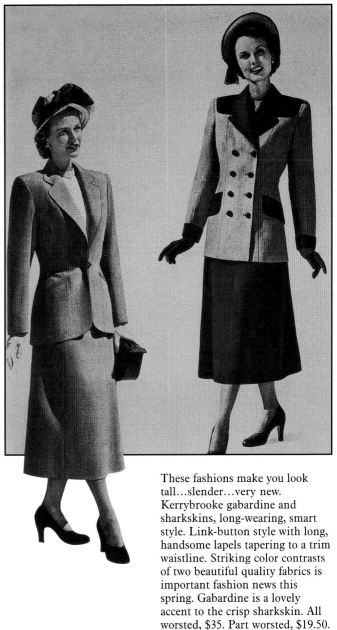

These fashions make you look tall…slender…very new. Kerrybrooke gabardine and sharkskins, long-wearing, smart style. Link-button style with long, handsome lapels tapering to a trim waistline. Striking color contrasts of two beautiful quality fabrics is important fashion news this spring. Gabardine is a lovely accent to the crisp sharkskin. All worsted, $35. Part worsted, $19.50. [$20-30] *Spring/summer 1949*

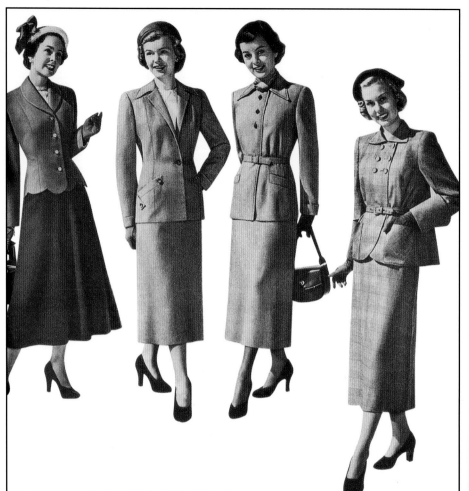

Ballerina Suit, wee-waisted jacket with scallops curving 'round the bottom. Jacket in light gray, emerald green, or bright red with a navy blue skirt. Spic-and-span sharkskin suit, perfect from desk to dates with the constant assurance of looking super-smart, in gray or brown mixture. Three-in-one suit, belted, half-belted, or swinging loose and free. Cavalier cuffs, rayon-lined, in brown or gray plaid. $17-22. [$20-30] *Spring/summer 1949*

Easy-to-launder women's work clothes. Sanforized fabrics for permanent fit. Tan poplin jackets, sateen lined or unlined. Cotton twill or sturdy gabardine slacks, in navy blue or dark brown. Smart, checked shirt in red, black, and white. Sanforized denim skirt or wraparound-style printed seersucker dress. Blue and white pincheck dress for extra working comfort. $2-6. [$5-10] *Spring/summer 1949*

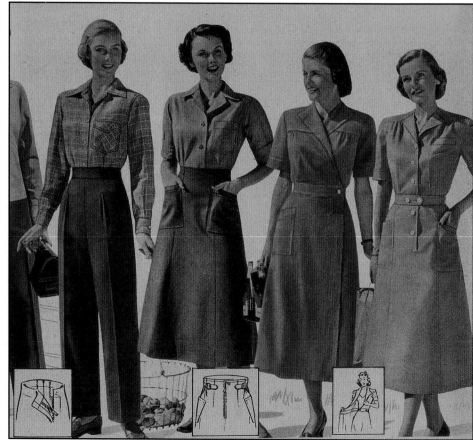

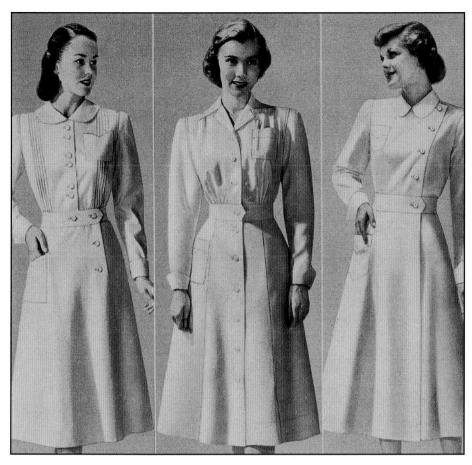

Kerrybrooke professional uniforms, in Sanforized broadcloth, two-ply poplin, or rayon sharkskin. Round collar with tucked front, buttons to waist. Convertible collar with pocket, stitched slot for thermometer, long or short sleeves. Smart, side-buttoned uniform with Peter Pan collar. $4-7. [$5-10] *Spring/summer 1949*

Superior quality uniforms for beauty parlor, factory, restaurant, laboratory, or home wear. A variety of styles, including button-front, coat style, zipper-front, or slipover dress that buttons to waist. Sanforized cotton with linen-like finish or Sanforized broadcloth, in white, blue, or green. $3-4. [$5-10] *Spring/summer 1949*

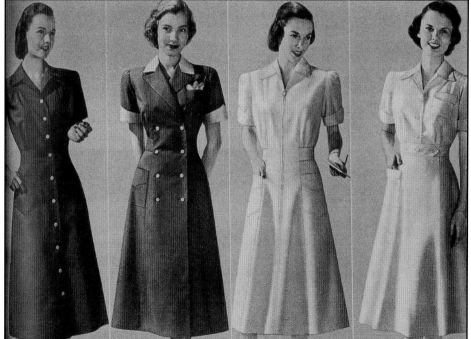

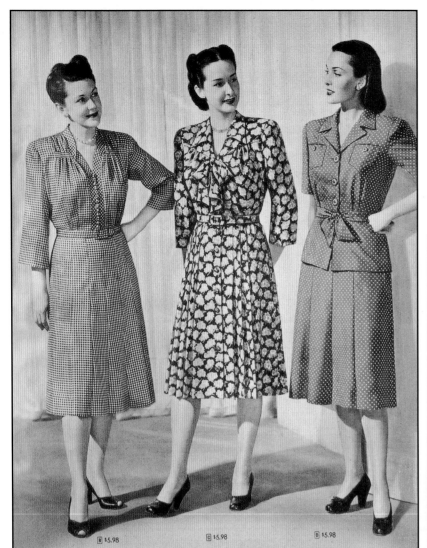

Casual

Kerrybrooke small check casual dress is crisp and fresh, in rayon crepe. Black and white, with soft shoulder shirring. Ever-popular button-front, colorful floral print in rayon crepe, styled in soft, dressmaker lines. Navy or royal blue ground, with pink, green, white, or gray flowers. Two-piece polka dot, so important in a woman's wardrobe…young and flattering, wear in all seasons. Navy Blue or dark green with white dots. $5.98 each. [$10-20] *Fall/winter 1946-1947*

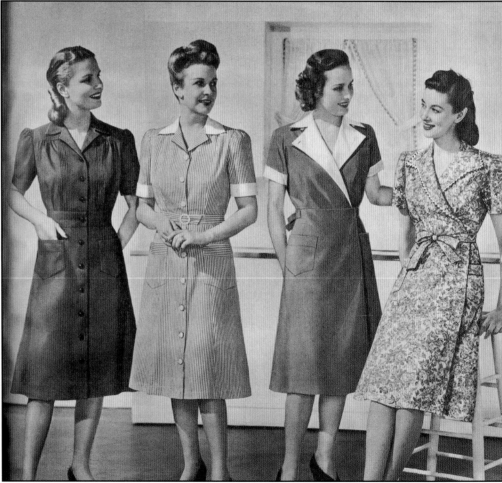

Button up or tie around…sturdy cotton work dresses in comfortable styles, for on the job or around the house. Button-front, solid reversible, or Magiwrap in posy print percale. $2-3. [$5-10] *Fall/winter 1946-1947*

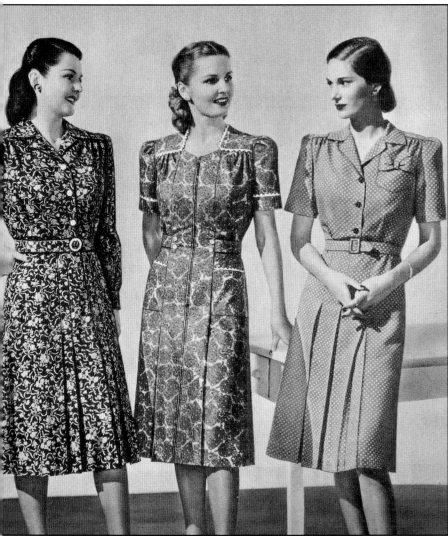

Trim and practical tub cottons for a woman's day. Long sleeve floral percale, convertible neckline, longer skirt, in navy or rose. Zipper-front flower percale, tie back belt. Medium blue or red background. Shirtwaist dress, gathered at shoulders and nipped in at waistlines by tiny darts. Polka dot print in good cotton-and-rayon fabric, in navy or rose. $3. [$5-15] *Fall/winter 1946-1947*

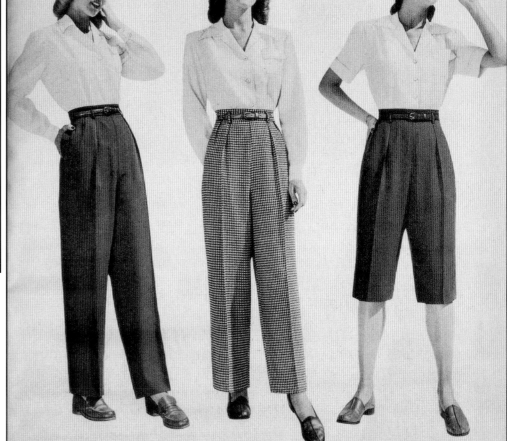

For smart, slim lines 'fore and aft…Kerrybrooke slacks and pedal pushers are a sure hit! All wool flannel slacks, in navy blue, dark brown, or black. Dapper checks for that smart, young boy look, part wool. Black and white check, or brown and white check. Pedal pushers, a hit fashion with the young crowd, famous Tacoma rayon. Navy blue, dark brown, or bright green. $4-7. [$20-30] *Spring/summer 1947*

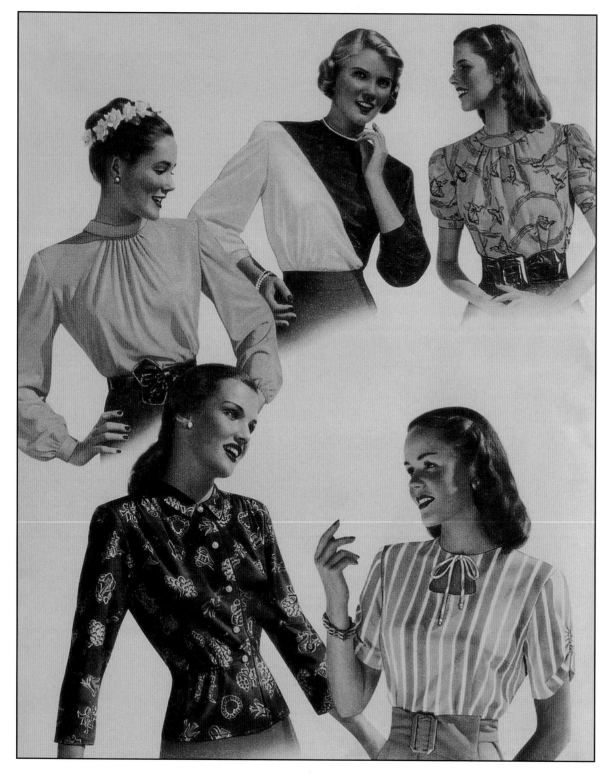

Costume blouses in colorful rayon jersey and shantung. New necklines, new prints, and new colors for the season. Turtleneck jersey in sleek, fine rayon, in white, pink, or light yellow. Half-black, half-white rayon jersey on a striking diagonal. Ballerina print rayon shantung with gay ballet dancers printed in black, on aqua, pink, yellow, or white ground. Rayon sweetheart print with hearts and lovebirds, on black or white ground. Sugar candy stripes, blend of pastels with becoming keyhole neckline with string bow. $4-5. [$15-30] *Spring/summer 1947*

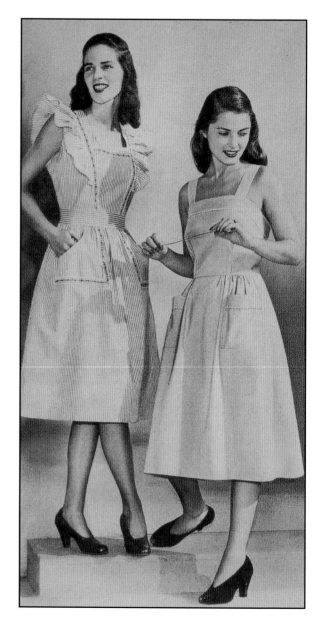

OPPOSITE PAGE, RIGHT -
Even the teakettle will whistle when you wear these around home! Ruffled sleeveless with fitted top and colorful peasant-style braid trim. Copen blue and white, or aqua green and white. Sunback dress of fine Sanforized chambray with full skirt and back buttons, in beige, pink, or medium blue. $3.39. [$5-15] *Spring/summer 1947*

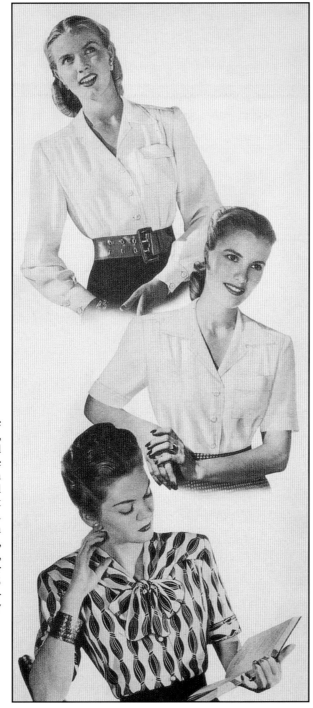

Famous Kerrybrooke shirt, known for its clean, smart lines. Collar shaped to lie flat, very fine stitching. Classic rayon crepe with slim, youthful lines. Club collar and short sleeves with cuffs in white. Women's rayon jersey with deep yoke and soft bow, becoming to fuller figures, in white and black, or aqua blue and white. $3-5 [$15-30] *Spring/summer 1947*

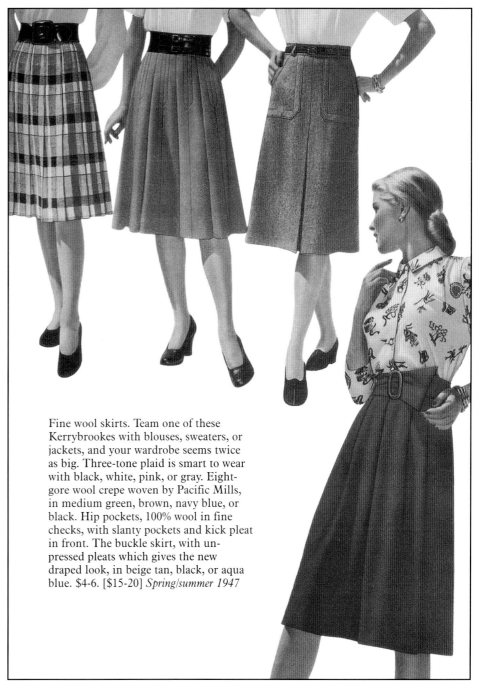

Fine wool skirts. Team one of these Kerrybrookes with blouses, sweaters, or jackets, and your wardrobe seems twice as big. Three-tone plaid is smart to wear with black, white, pink, or gray. Eight-gore wool crepe woven by Pacific Mills, in medium green, brown, navy blue, or black. Hip pockets, 100% wool in fine checks, with slanty pockets and kick pleat in front. The buckle skirt, with un-pressed pleats which gives the new draped look, in beige tan, black, or aqua blue. $4-6. [$15-20] *Spring/summer 1947*

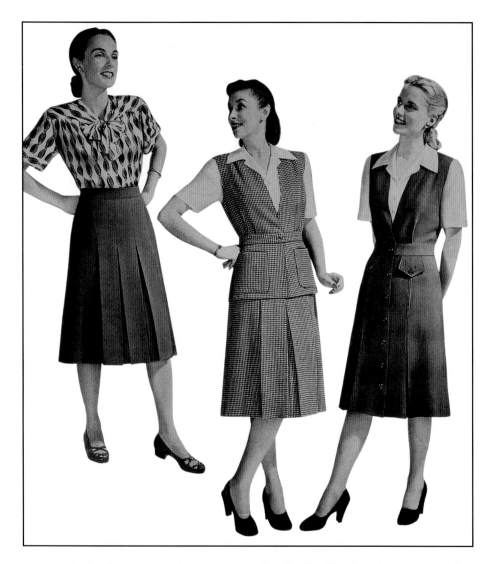

Sports clothes for women…trim, young, and slimming. Pacific all wool crepe skirt with three box pleats in front and back, in dark brown, black, or navy blue. Checked two-piece jerkin outfit, belted waistline with one-button closing, in black and white check. One-piece jumper, 78% spun rayon, 22% wool, becoming to women's figures, in navy, medium brown, or deep aqua blue. $4-8. [$10-15] *Spring/summer 1947*

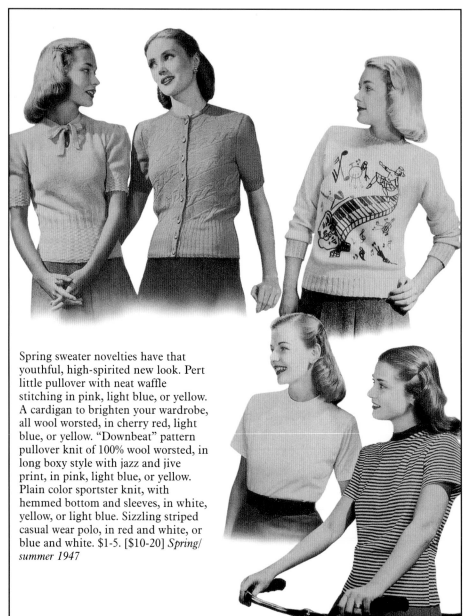

Spring sweater novelties have that youthful, high-spirited new look. Pert little pullover with neat waffle stitching in pink, light blue, or yellow. A cardigan to brighten your wardrobe, all wool worsted, in cherry red, light blue, or yellow. "Downbeat" pattern pullover knit of 100% wool worsted, in long boxy style with jazz and jive print, in pink, light blue, or yellow. Plain color sportster knit, with hemmed bottom and sleeves, in white, yellow, or light blue. Sizzling striped casual wear polo, in red and white, or blue and white. $1-5. [$10-20] *Spring/summer 1947*

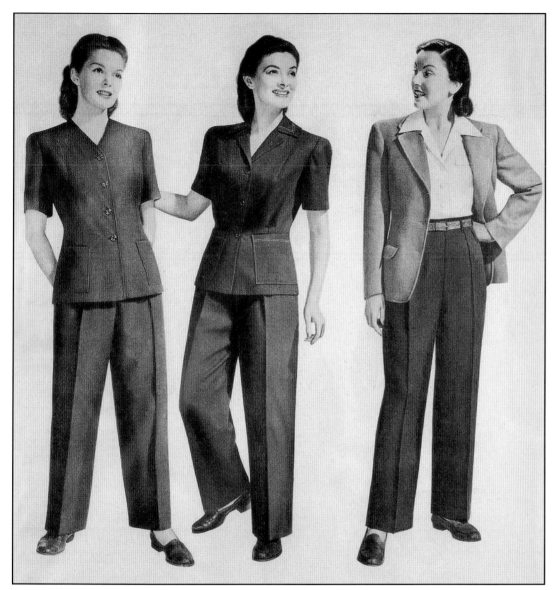

Sporty suits, good for work or play. Rayon shantung slack suit with cardigan-type jacket, in navy blue, brown, or black. Slack suit of Sanforized cotton twill, slenderizing dark colors with contrasting saddle stitching, in navy blue or brown. Handsome all wool jacket in domestic Shetland-type tweed, in navy blue, brown, or black. $6-10. [$15-25] *Fall/winter 1948*

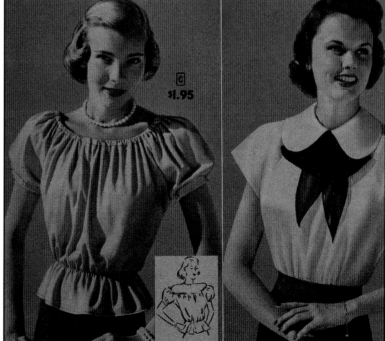

New fashions in blousettes. Rayon jersey sheds wrinkles and adds sparkle to suits, in black, medium blue, or light pink ground. Youthful blousette in a shirred back style with new pointed collar, in black, brown, light pink, or red. Shirred neckline to wear for daytime, or off-the-shoulder for parties, in white, red, Kelly green, or medium blue. Windsor bow in crisp, shining rayon sharkskin, nice fitting shirred waistline, in white with a black bow. $2-3. [$10-20] *Fall/winter 1948*

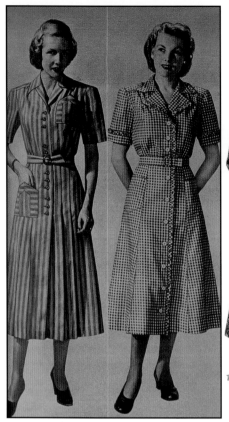

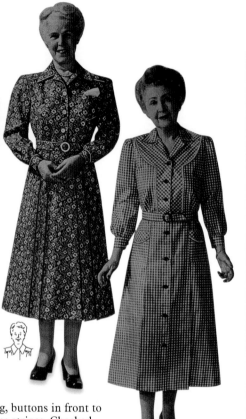

Sanforized chambray stripes are slenderizing, buttons in front to the hipline. Gray and yellow, or gray and rose stripes. Checked percale with neat self ruffles, button-front softened by full ruffles of self fabric, in brown and white, blue and white, or green and white. Longer skirts made with Kerrybrooke cottons for the gracious lady, with small flowers on navy or rose in a year-round percale, or a check percale with white cotton lace trim in green, blue, or lavender with white. $3-5. [$10-20] *Fall/winter 1948*

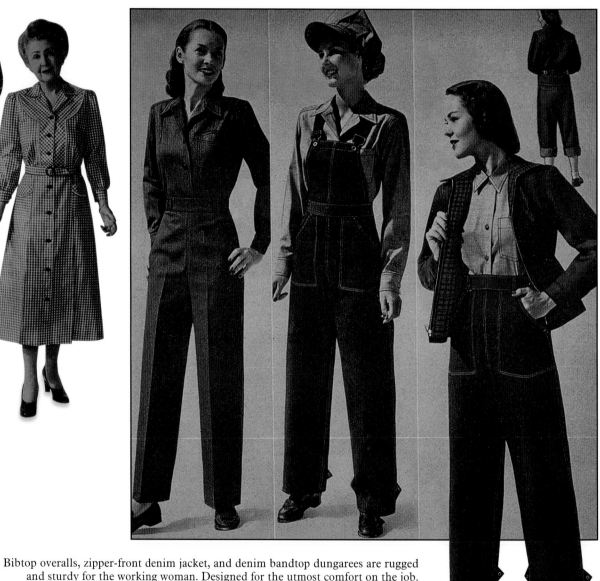

Bibtop overalls, zipper-front denim jacket, and denim bandtop dungarees are rugged and sturdy for the working woman. Designed for the utmost comfort on the job. Sanforized cotton fabrics won't shrink over 1%! All in denim blue, some in Oxford gray. Shirts, $1-2. Slacks and dungarees, $2-3. Overalls, $2-3. [$30-50] *Fall/winter 1948*

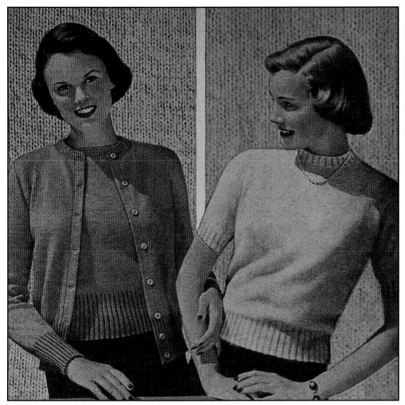

Aristocrat of sweater yarns…25% smooth, cloud-light cashmere blended with 75% fine virgin zephyr wool, long sleeve cardigan or short sleeve pullover, smart natural color. 50% angora, 50% zephyr wool…the softest, fluffiest, and loveliest of luxury sweaters. Classic short sleeve pullover style tops everything smartly. Fitted cardigan, styled to flatter the mature figure, beautifully knit in long-wearing, 100% wool worsted yarns to keep you snug in chilly weather. $3-7. [$25-40] *Fall/winter 1948*

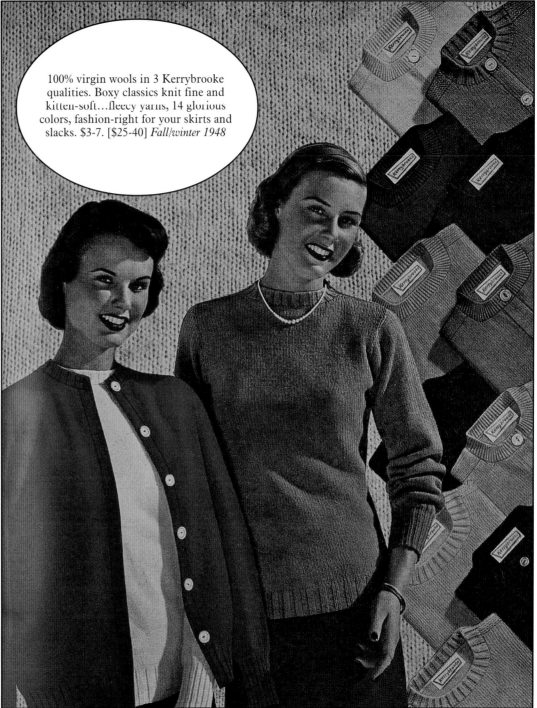

100% virgin wools in 3 Kerrybrooke qualities. Boxy classics knit fine and kitten-soft…fleecy yarns, 14 glorious colors, fashion-right for your skirts and slacks. $3-7. [$25-40] *Fall/winter 1948*

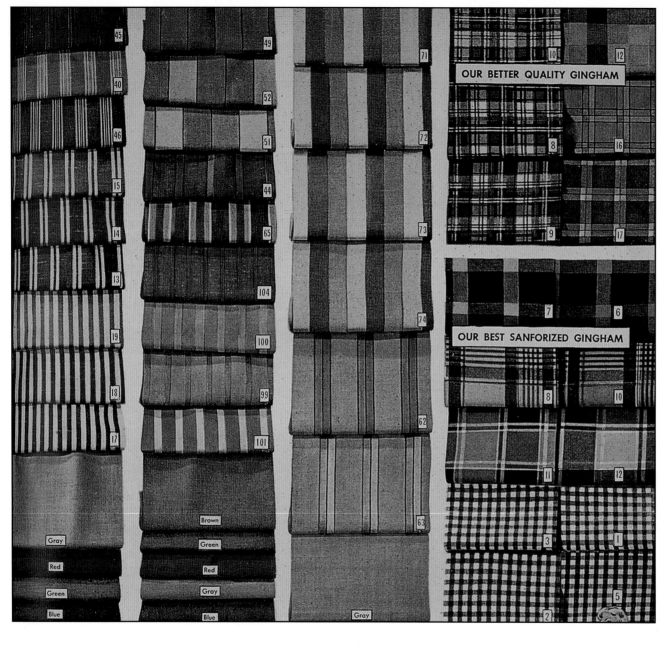

OUR BETTER QUALITY GINGHAM

OUR BEST SANFORIZED GINGHAM

Gray
Red
Green
Blue

Brown
Green
Red
Gray
Blue

Gray

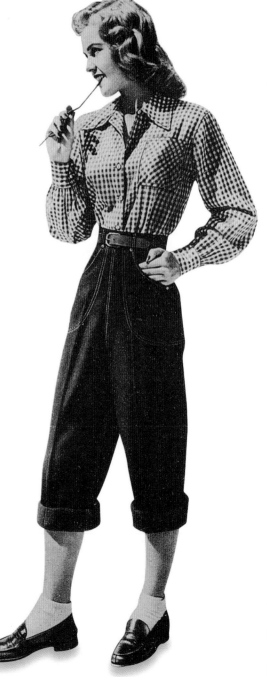

Sanforized chambrays and ginghams for every use. Long-wearing, durable fabrics find hundreds of year-round uses in the family wardrobe and the household. From 60¢ a yard. [$1/yard] *Fall/winter 1948*

Cold weather Kerrybrookes, warmly lined and very practical. Two-piece gabardine outfit, cotton poplin jacket, whole suit lined with cotton kasha, water repellent. Black with gray, or navy blue with red. $16. Heavy twenty-four-ounce melton cloth slacks, 100% reprocessed wool lined with kasha. Navy blue, dark brown, dark green. $6-7. Sanforized denim dungarees, strong double needle stitching in contrasting colors. Navy blue, barn red, or light blue. $2. [$15-$25] *Fall/winter 1948*

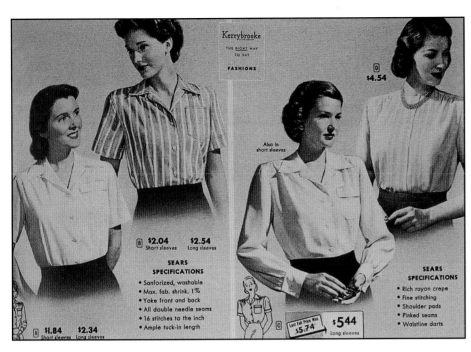

Sanforized cotton Kerrybrooke shirts, durable washfast. White, pastels, or stripes. Blouses with slim lines for figure flattery, cut amply full with roomy armholes. Yellow, gray, white, pink, or light blue. $2-5. [$15-20] *Spring/summer 1949*

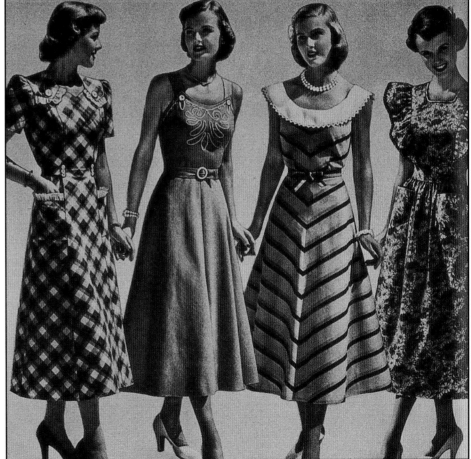

Crisp, washable cottons, gay new prints, easy fitting. Budget cottons for all day long, generously cut. Fresh, bright colors, in stripes, plaids, and solids. Pinafore pretties are carefree young flatterers for workday comfort, home, and glamour in the sun! Pinks, browns, blues, grays, and greens, with assorted floral prints. $3-4. [$15-20] *Spring/summer 1949*

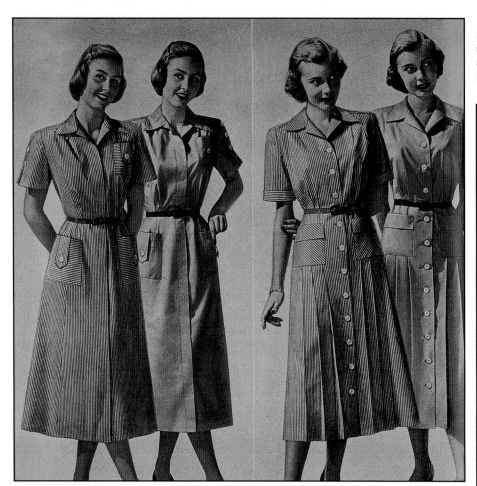

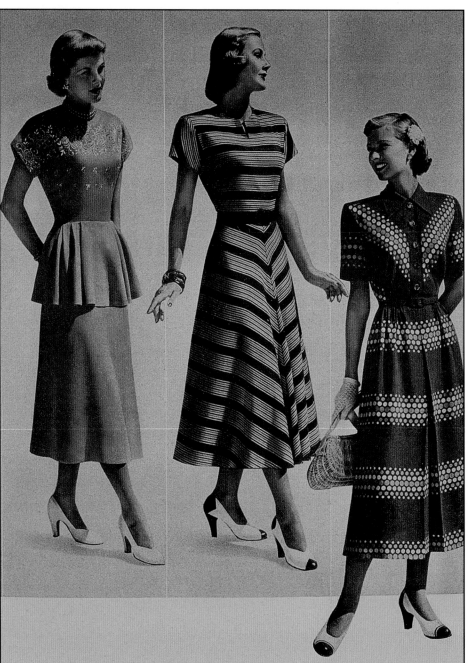

Smart, clean-cut, washable Kerrybrooke cottons, in four striped patterns and four lovely solid pastels. Hems are two inches deep, giving ample allowance for lengthening. Pink, aqua green, lavender, gray solids, red, blue, brown, and green with white stripes. $5-6. [$10-20] *Spring/summer 1949*

Easy-to-wash spun rayon with good tailoring and finishing. Handsome embroidery, candy stripes, and colorful coin dot stripes, in slim or full skirt styles. Very smart and casual. Lilac, coral rose, medium gray, aqua blue, or multicolored stripes. $5-7. [$10-15] *Spring/summer 1949*

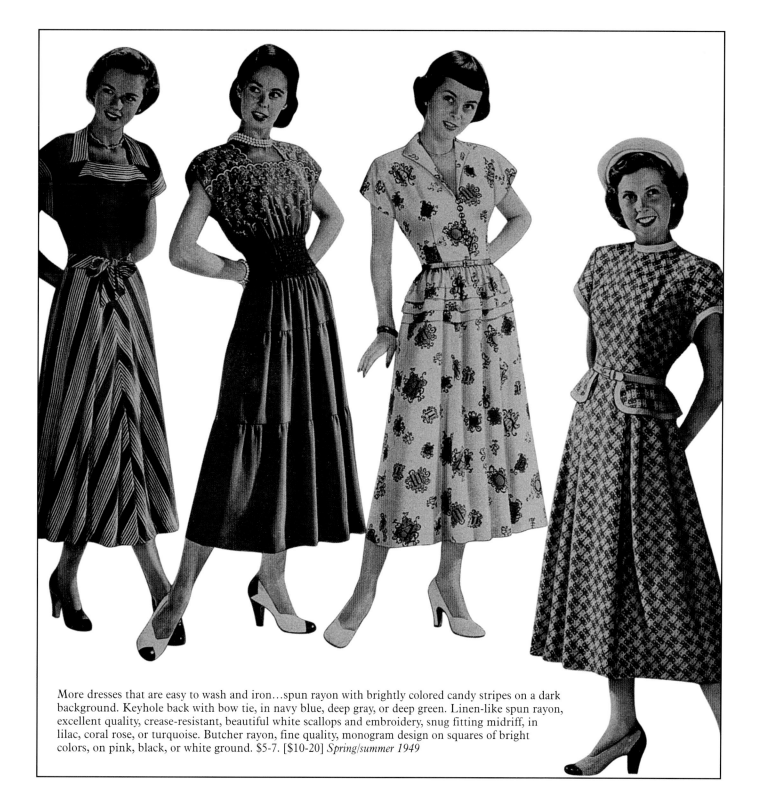

More dresses that are easy to wash and iron…spun rayon with brightly colored candy stripes on a dark background. Keyhole back with bow tie, in navy blue, deep gray, or deep green. Linen-like spun rayon, excellent quality, crease-resistant, beautiful white scallops and embroidery, snug fitting midriff, in lilac, coral rose, or turquoise. Butcher rayon, fine quality, monogram design on squares of bright colors, on pink, black, or white ground. $5-7. [$10-20] *Spring/summer 1949*

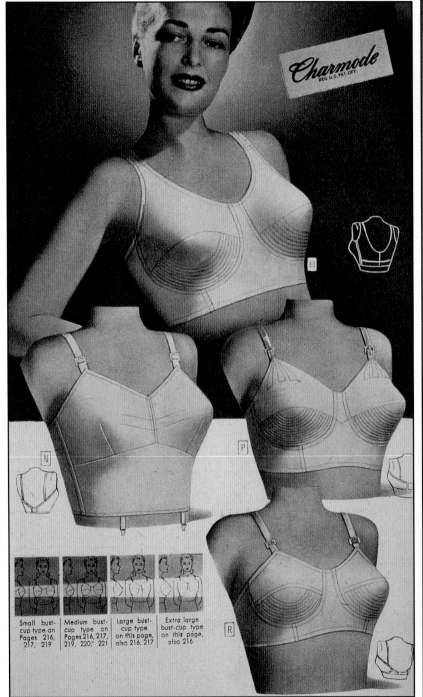

Charmode
REG U.S. PAT. OFF.

| Small bust-cup type on Pages 216, 217, 219 | Medium bust-cup type on Pages 216, 217, 219, 220," 221 | Large bust-cup type on this page, also 216, 217 | Extra large bust-cup type on this page, also 216 |

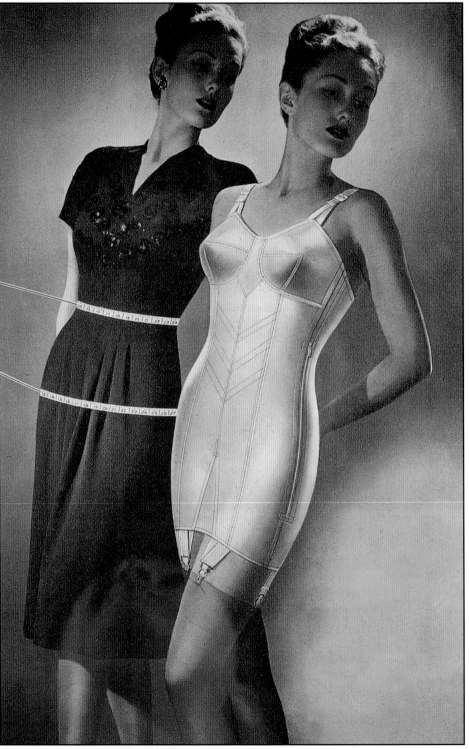

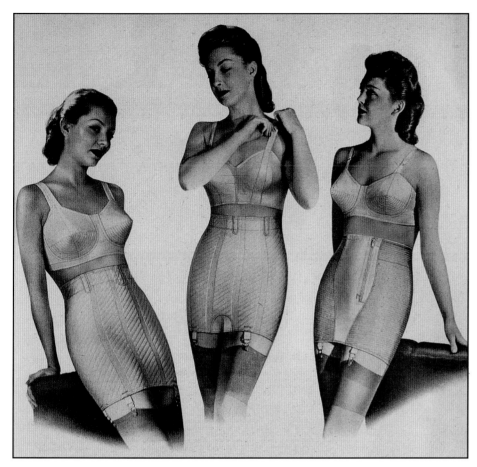

Slenderizing Charmode garments made of wonderful two-way stretch all-elastic, figure-trimming. Panty girdle and overlay panel tummy control, four elastic garters, all garments in nude color. $4-5. [$15-20] *Fall/winter 1946-1947*

Flater-ees quality vests, briefs, and panties, in blush color wisps of soft, caressingly smooth cotton, firmly knit for skin-smooth fit. 40¢-50¢. [$5] *Fall/winter 1947*

OPPOSITE PAGE

LEFT · Charmode bras for large bust-cup sizes. In rayon-cotton mix or just cotton, pale flesh pink color. $1-3. [$5-10] *Fall/winter 1946-1947*

RIGHT · Glamorous Charmode all-in-one. A fashion-right silhouette is guaranteed with this beautiful foundation. Made of shimmering rayon and cotton satin with bust highly accentuated and cotton lined. $8.50. [$10-15] *Fall/winter 1946-1947*

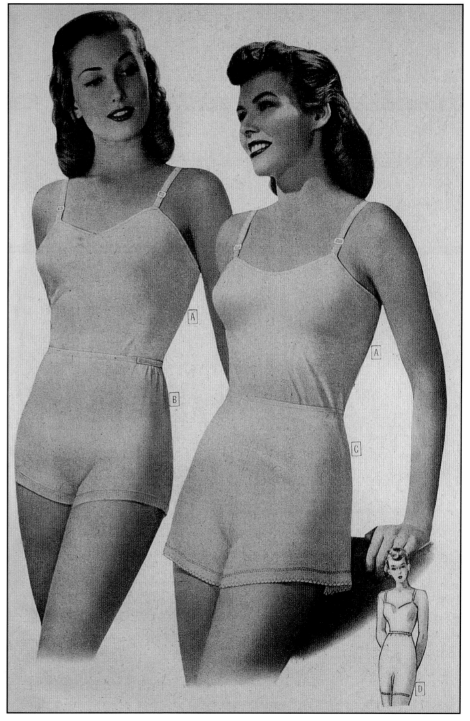

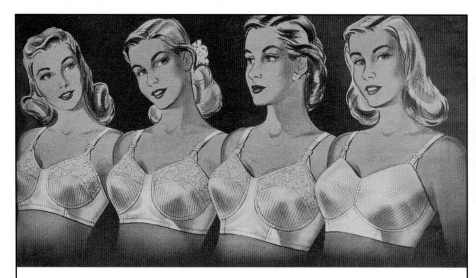

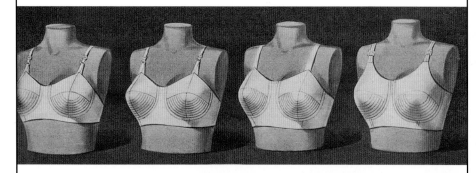

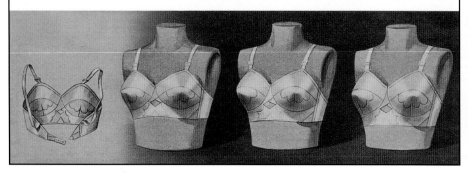

Charmode "Underlift" bras, with famous three-way strap control "Underlift" feature to create a lovely bustline. Stretchable rayon and firmer cotton styles, in pale flesh pink. Cordtex bras have "the beauty lift that lasts." Inserts give more support where most needed, in three bust-cup sizes. $1-4. [$5-10] *Spring/summer 1947*

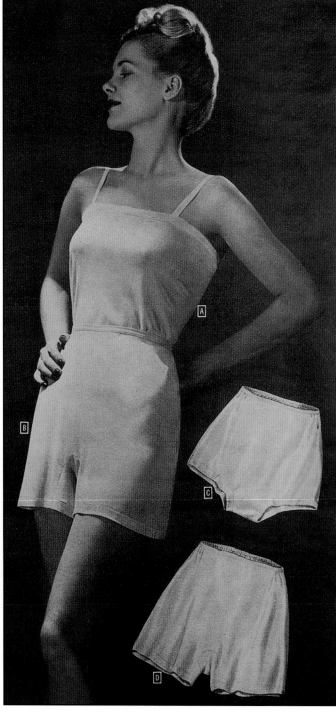

Smart women everywhere say it's the soft, long-wearing fabric, the easy, comfortable fit, and the simple tailored styles that make Sears knit rayons a number one underwear choice! Flare leg panty, band leg brief, or band leg panty, along with tearose pink soft vest, for maximum comfort. 50¢-60¢. [$5] *Spring/summer 1947*

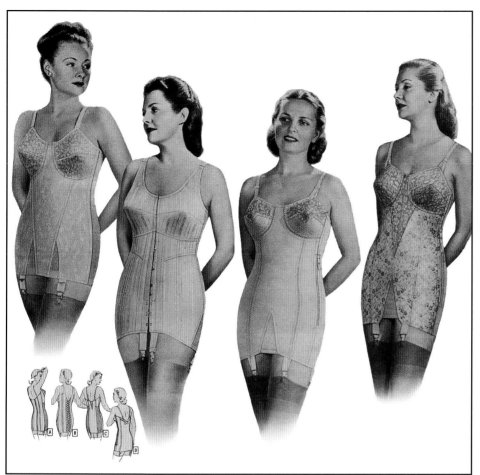

All-in-one foundations by Charmode give comfortable, allover support to the fuller figure. Styles custom tailored for different body types, short, tall, fuller…each with a slimming, trimming effect. $2-4. [$10-15] *Spring/summer 1947*

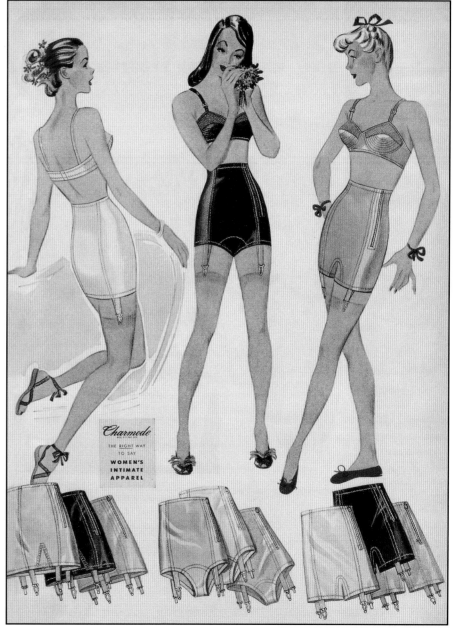

You'll thrill over the luxurious, shimmering beauty of these smartly designed Charmode foundation garments and lovely brassieres. Lustrous all-elastic synthetic rubber woven with rayon and cotton for extra comfort and stretch. In pale flesh pink, black, white, or pale blue. Entirely boneless corsetry with fagoted front for straight to average hip figure. $6. Marvelous wearing comfort brassiere for medium bust-cup. $3. [$5-10] *Spring/summer 1947*

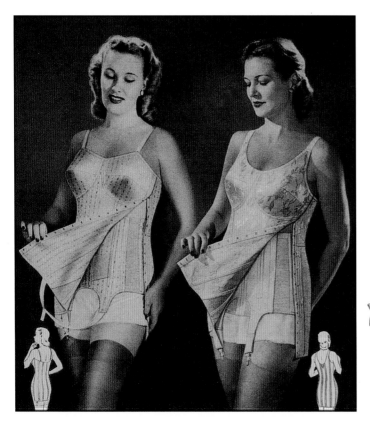

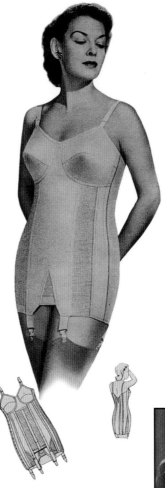

These Charmode all-in-ones provide extra abdominal control for the fuller figure. Designed with or without inner belts for average to full hip figures. Well-boned inner belt and full length cotton elastic panels for smooth, slenderizing support. Fine quality rayon, striped cotton fabric, or high grade preshrunk brocaded cotton and rayon batiste, in nude. $4-7. [$10-15] *Spring/summer 1947*

Sears Scientific Supports for specific figure needs give balanced body support and utmost comfort. Sturdy cotton and patented designs help relieve fatigue, support the abdomen, and improve posture. "Nulife" braces and belts, in white. $1-$3. Charmode "Slack Sash," in flesh pink. $3. [$5-10] *Spring/summer 1947*

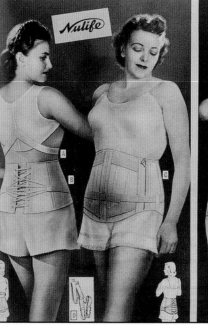

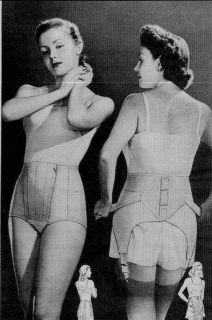

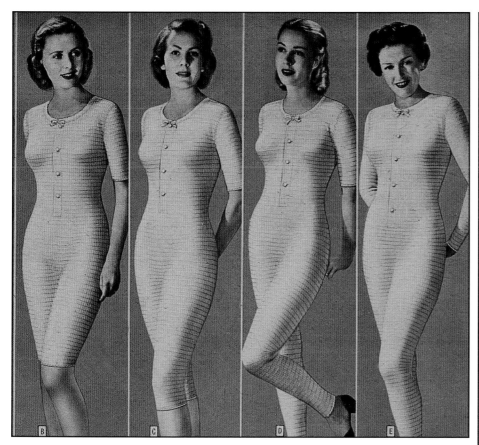

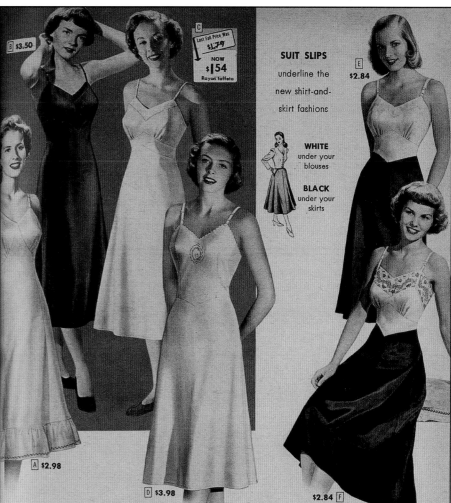

SUIT SLIPS
underline the
new shirt-and-
skirt fashions

E
$2.84

WHITE
under your
blouses

BLACK
under your
skirts

A $2.98

D $3.98

$2.84 F

Charmode part wool and all wool union suits…five toasty-warm styles and four qualities to fit your every need. Rib knit in extrafine gauge to stretch easily as you move. Skillfully narrowed and shaped in at the waist for trim fit, in cream. $2-7. [$10-15] *Fall/winter 1948*

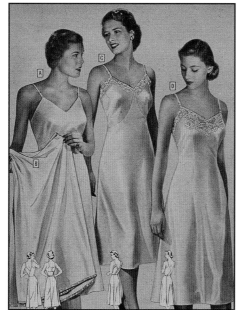

Tailored slips in rayon crepes and taffetas…deftly fitted for smooth lines and firmly sewn for long wear. Different styles feature adjustable straps and a variety of colors. $2-4. Suit slips with white tailored bodices and black biased skirts. Extra "swish" under your skirts! $3. [$5-15] *Spring/summer 1949*

Maternity slips…trimmed or tailored styles for the mother-to-be, with deep overlaps for easy adjustment. Lovely and luxurious to wear under suits or dresses. Hand washable cotton and rayon flat crepe with Alencon-type cotton lace, in white or tearose. $2-5. [$10-15] *Fall/winter 1948*

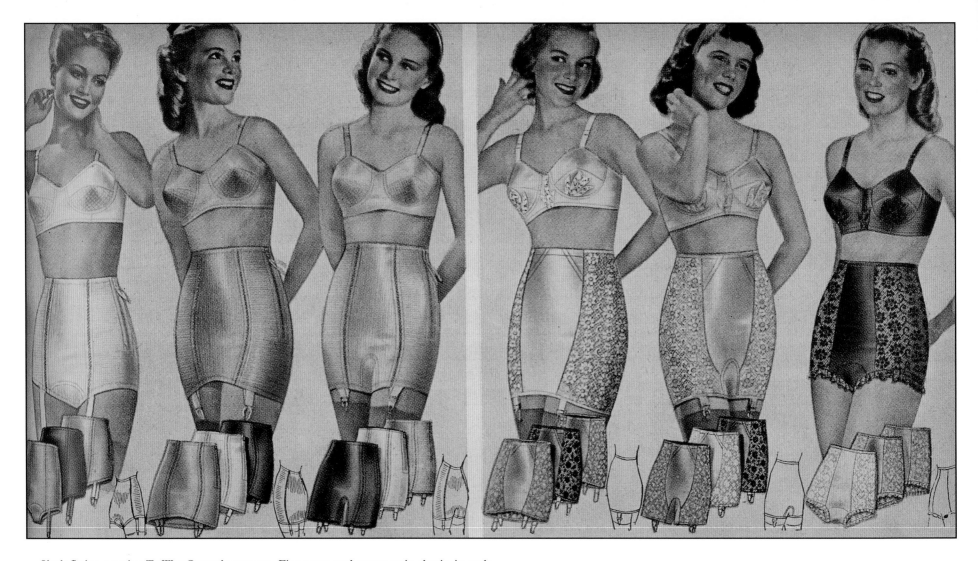

Sleek-fitting genuine Tu-Way Control garments. Fine rayon and cotton satin elastic, in nude, white, pale blue, and black. Famous maker design with fagoted seams in front and back, boneless. $5. Lace elastic girdles, panty girdles, and briefs are pretty, dainty, and popular, in white, nude, pale blue, and black. $3-4. Matching bras, $2. [$5-10] *Fall/winter 1948*

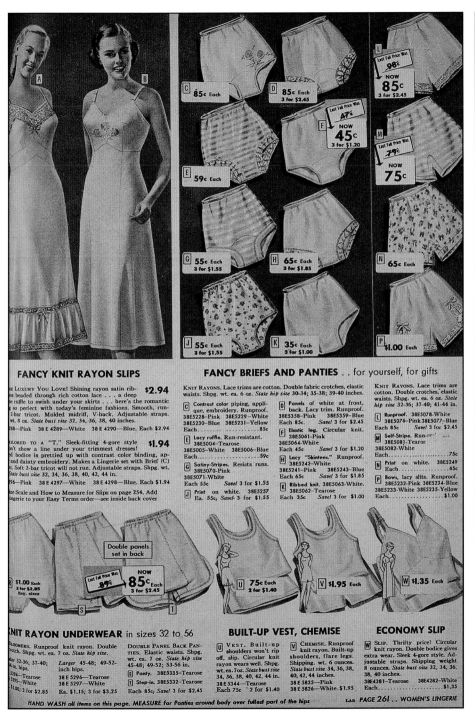

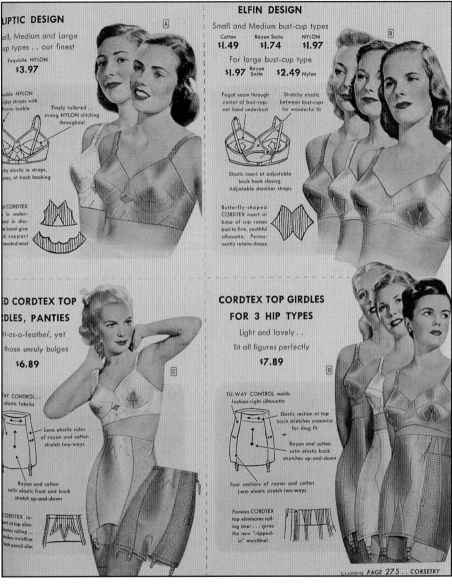

Truly remarkable…this magic ribbed rayon-and-cotton fabric provides firm uplift in a bra—a non-roll top on a girdle…not only when your garment is new, but always! Charmode's famous Cordtex stays firm after repeated launderings. Nylon, cotton, and rayon satin bras, in nude, white, and blue. $1.50-4. Rayon and cotton girdles make waistlines look pencil-slim, in nude or white. $7-8. [$5-10] *Spring/summer 1949*

Fancy briefs and panties…for yourself or for gifts. In knit rayons with cotton lace trims, double crotches, and elastic waists. Wide variety of colors and styles. 60¢-$1. [$5-10] *Spring/summer 1949*

Outerwear

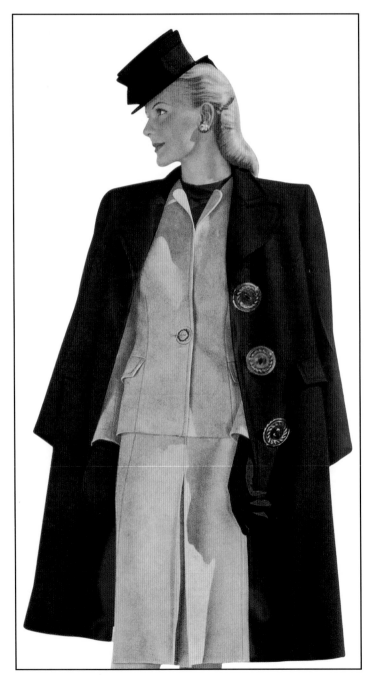

In soft-finish virgin wool, with rich, smooth weave, the skillful tailoring that distinguishes Kerrybrookes comes to you in a stylish, superbly classic boy coat. Perfect to pair with your favorite suit. In royal blue or medium brown. $35. [$50-100] *Fall/winter 1946-1947*

Flange shoulders and big buttons on a neat and easy coat, in smart, soft-finish wool. Black for the coat, daylight color for a suit underneath, with each taking on fashion's newest details to make their separate lives more interesting. Suit in rosy red, royal blue, or medium gray. Coat or suit, $35. [$30-40] *Fall/winter 1946-1947*

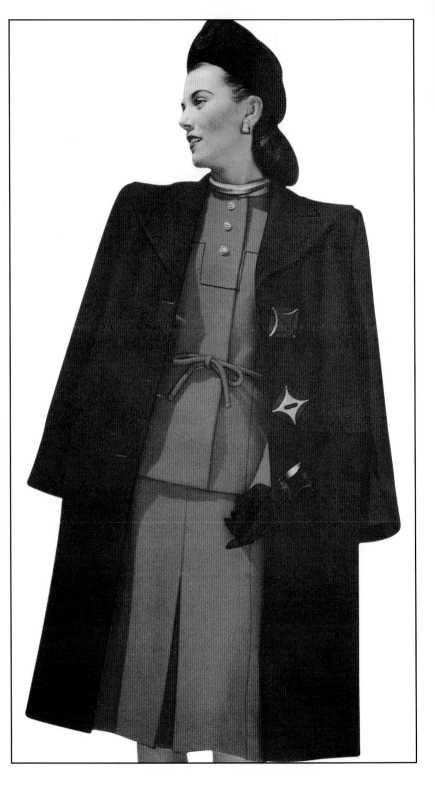

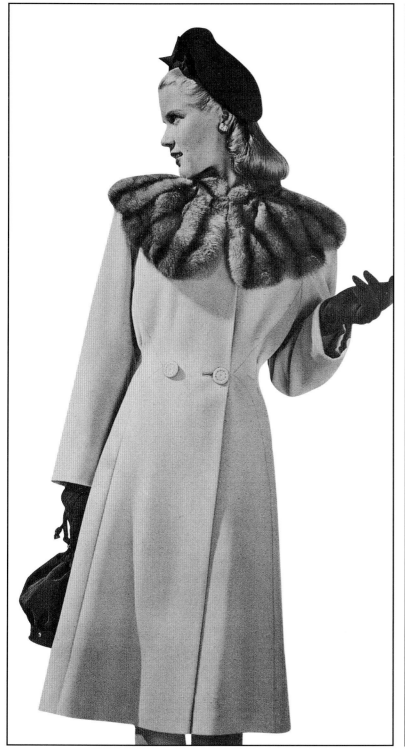

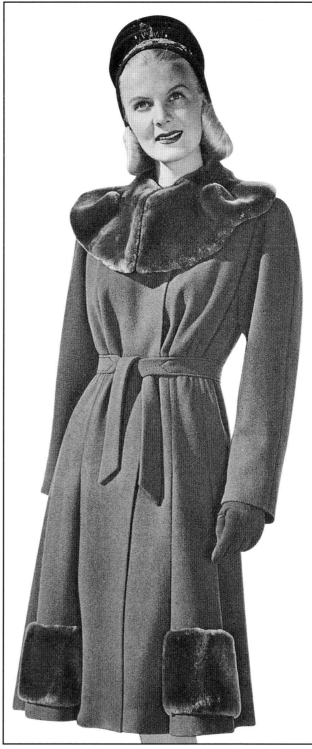

LEFT · Ripple-fold fur collar adds a luxury touch to the twin-buttoned coat with shapely waistline. New, fuller sleeves with a choice of two fashionable furs: silver blue-dyed Russian squirrel, or beaver-dyed Conley collar. In black, dark brown, medium blue, or winter white (light gray). $45, $60. [$45-$70] *Fall/winter 1946-1947*

RIGHT · Fur lavished and tautly tied at the waistline…with swingy fur-hemmed skirt panels and artful gathers. Beaver-dyed mouton lamb or Coney trimming, this coat will keep you warm in the bitterest of winters. Rich, suede-soft pure wool, in dark brown, medium green, black, or royal blue. $40-50. [$45-70] *Fall/winter 1946-1947*

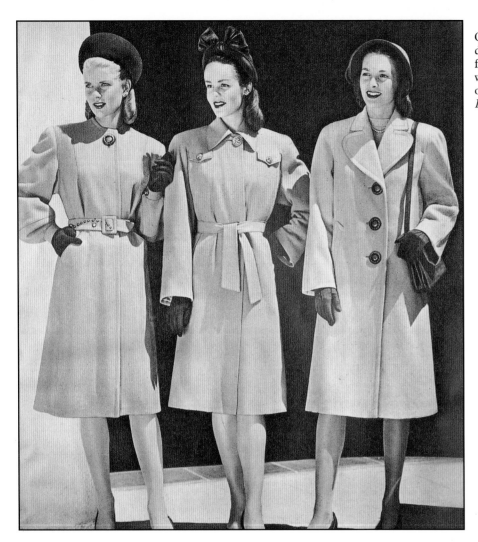

Glitter belt coat in rich, suede-soft wool bells its sleeves smartly. Rayon-lined, in black, dark brown, medium green, or medium blue. The velvety, all wool, tied-in-tight coat features fashion's new neck-buttoning and drops two smart flaps from well-set shoulders, in winter white, dark brown, medium green, and royal blue. Timeless boy coat, full cut for over suit wear, in black, dark brown, winter white, or medium blue. $23. [$20-30] *Fall/winter 1946-1947*

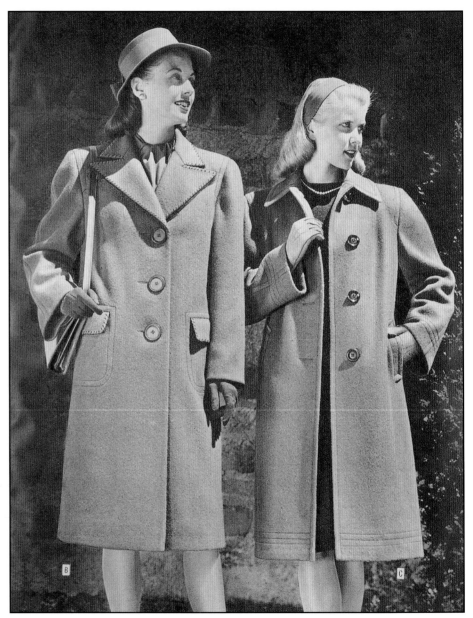

Knit back fleece coat, loomed and wear-tested, has pure wool face, cotton back, and wind-defying close threaded weave. Whipstitched boy coat with huge pockets and back vent pleat, in dark brown, medium blue, medium gray, or light soft green. The Balmacaan, go-with-everything coat with smartly convertible collar and deep armholes, in dark brown, medium blue, medium gray, or black. $23.50. [$20-30] *Fall/winter 1946/1947*

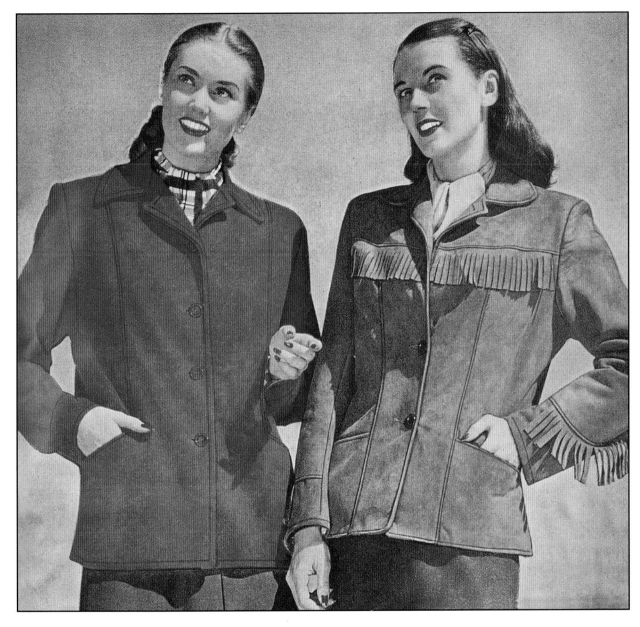

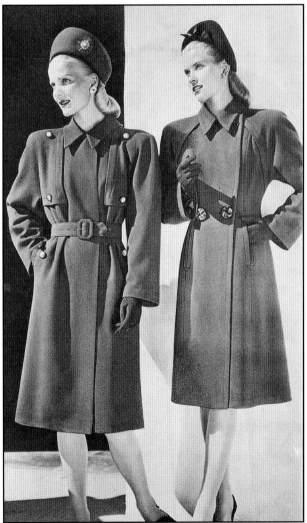

Jackets in glowing suede and capeskin with plaid linings. Boxy leather jacket with wing-type sleeves and snug-buttoned cuff, in red, green, or tan suede, and medium brown capeskin. Ranch-style jacket, back from last season. Soft leather, fringed all across the front, back, and part way up the sleeves, in medium green, tan, or red suede, and medium brown capeskin. $17-19. [$35-60] *Fall/winter 1946-1947*

Dressed-up winter coats cut generously in soft-touch woolens, with waistlines smartly belted, buttoned, or left alone. Bolero-effect coat with fashionable shoulder-into-sleeve treatment, in black, dark brown, wine red, or winter white (light gray). Twin-button coat with new winged sleeves, in royal blue, dark brown, medium green, or winter white. $23, $30. [$30-55] *Fall/winter 1946-1947*

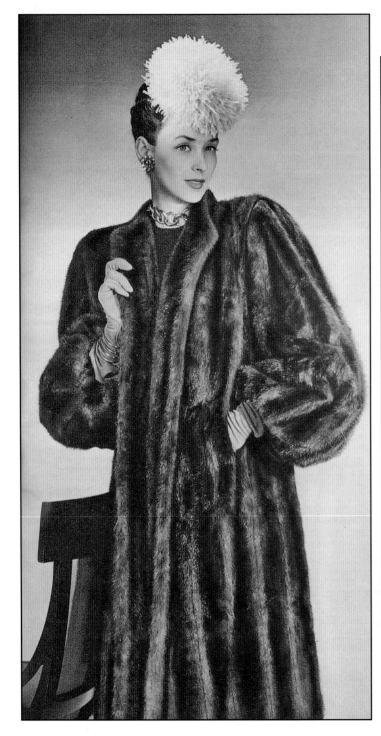

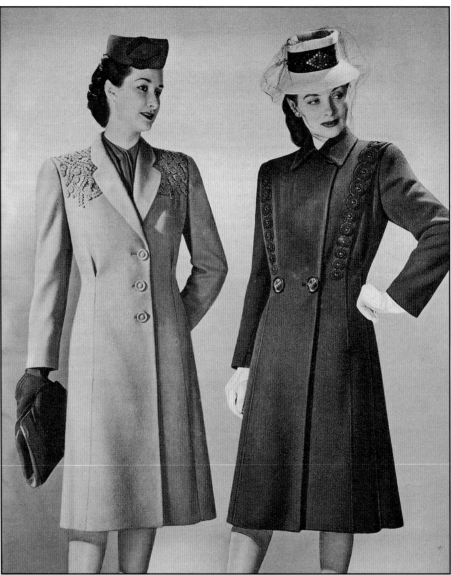

This slim-fitted coat with a softly rounded collar is youthful and flattering. Fashionable rococo embroidery enhances smart shoulders. Black, medium green, or medium blue. Twin-button coat in suede-soft all wool features embroidery sparked with jet-like centers adorning a tapering flange. Black, dark brown, or medium blue. $30, $35. [$10-20] *Fall/winter 1946-1947*

Hollander Mink-blended Northern Muskrat tuxedo coat. Ballooning sleeves, flange shoulders, and fine quality rayon lining. All choice back pelts, full-furred and silky. $300. [$75-100] *Fall/winter 1946-1947*

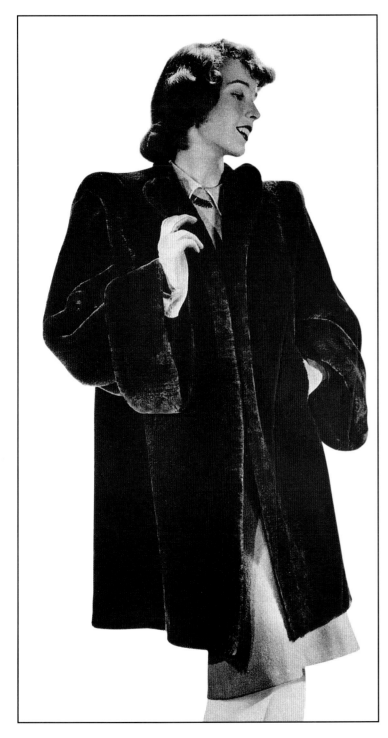

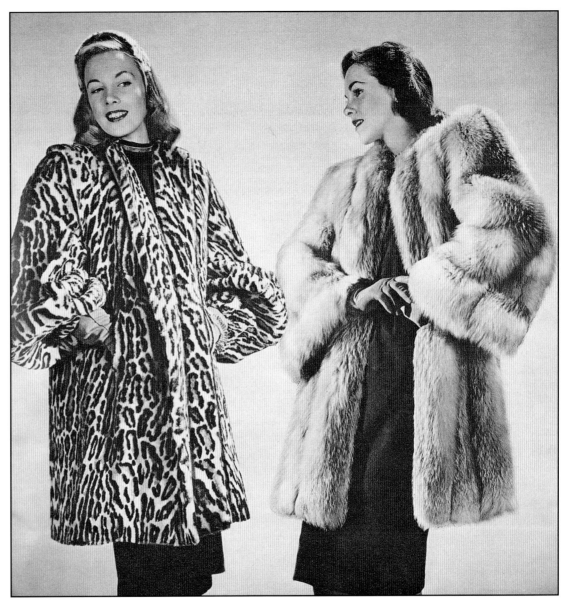

Dark ocelot markings on sheared alpine lamb, swingy tuxedo style with rich velvety finish. $90. Red fox greatcoat, vertically worked fur for beautiful full-blown look, rayon-lined. $125. [$50] *Fall/winter 1946-1947*

Beaver-dyed mouton lamb tuxedo coat, a swingy thirty-six incher with full sleeves and cardigan neck with wing lapels. Buttons high when cold winds blow, in beaver brown. $125. [$50] *Fall/winter 1946-1947*

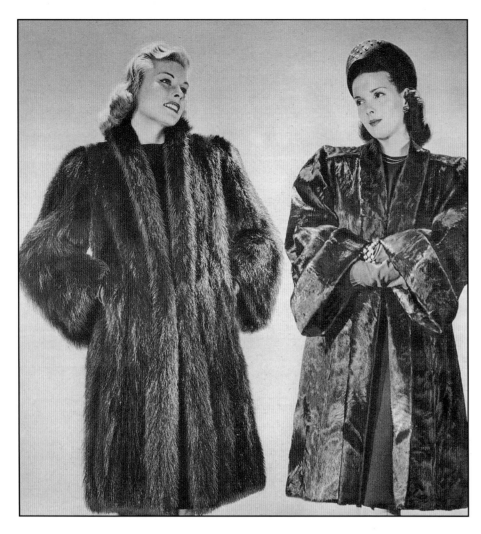

Dyed skunk, a beautiful glistening black. Collar rolls softly, sleeves newly wide. Dyed Russian pony, durable, richly moiré marked, dyed deep black with a great life and luster. $130, $125. [$50-75] *Fall/winter 1946-1947*

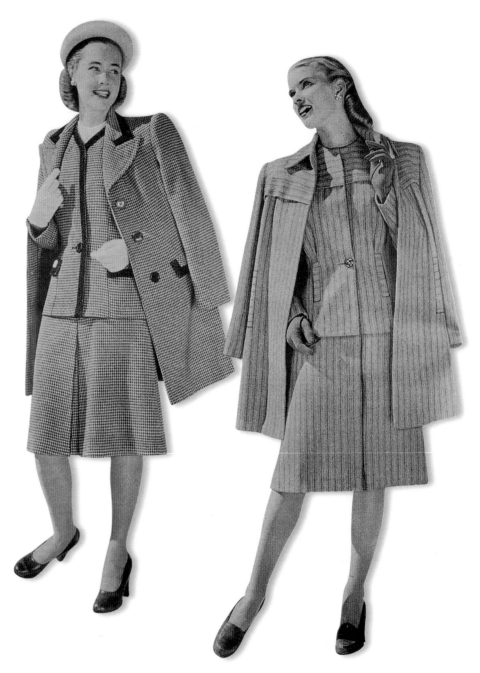

These shortcoats have a big fashion future! Checks, nice clear ones, in shape-holding all wool. Young and boxy, this coat's perky lapels peak and it's pockets flap to match those of the cardigan suit beneath it. Striped menswear flannel is spring's "number one" pure wool fabric. Clear stripes, worked for good figure line. Cleverly paired with matching suit. $17. [$25-40] *Spring/summer 1947*

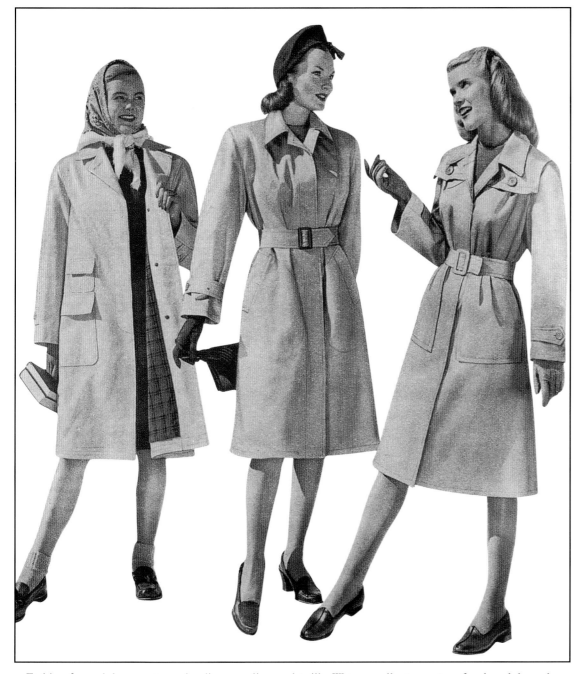

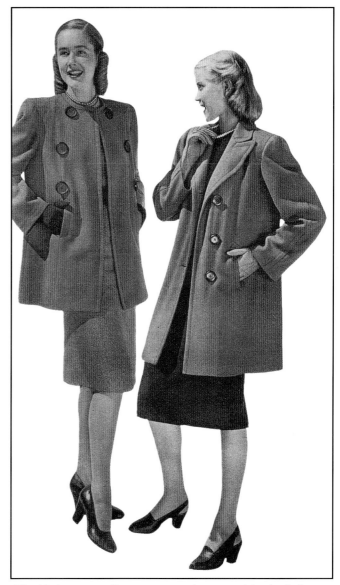

Fashion-favored dress coats…gabardines, poplins, and twills. Water-repellent, smart-surfaced, and dependable. All styles in medium tan, black, or navy blue. $7-12. [$20-30] *Spring/summer 1947*

The big-button cardigan, a snappy shortcoat with a back that flips out smartly in rippling flare, in medium blue, Kelly green, and coral. The snipped boy coat, a neat thirty-three inches, with jaunty peaked lapel collar or three nice big buttons. Toss over everything you own from slacks to dresses, in medium blue, medium brown, or Kelly green. $12-13. [$25-40] *Spring/summer 1947*

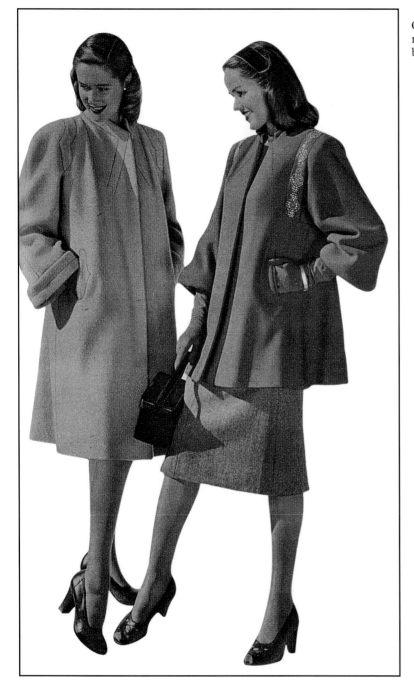

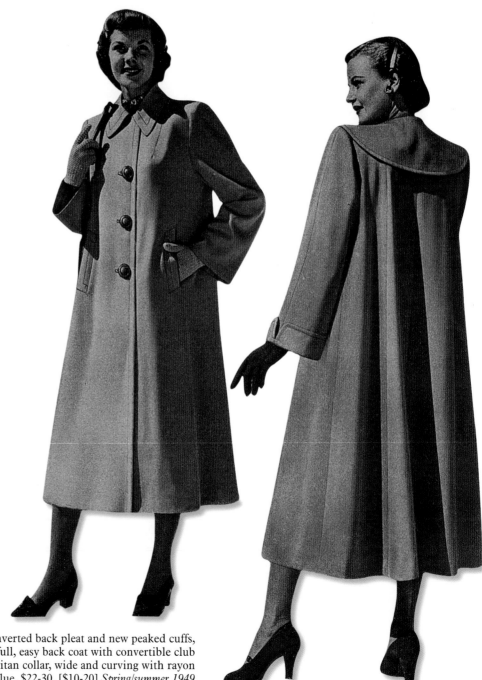

Casual coats look lavish, especially Kerrybrookes. Glitter thread, beautiful braid stitching, gleaming nailheads, in flare-back or ripple-back styles. Fluffy all wool fleece, in Kelly green, light gray, medium blue, brown, or black. $25. [$10-20] *Spring/summer 1947*

Flare-backs in rich gabardine or covert. A full-flowing style, deep inverted back pleat and new peaked cuffs, in emerald green, medium gray, black, or navy blue. Neatly tailored, full, easy back coat with convertible club collar, in emerald green, medium gray, coral red, or bright red. Puritan collar, wide and curving with rayon tie, in emerald green, medium gray, or navy blue. $22-30. [$10-20] *Spring/summer 1949*

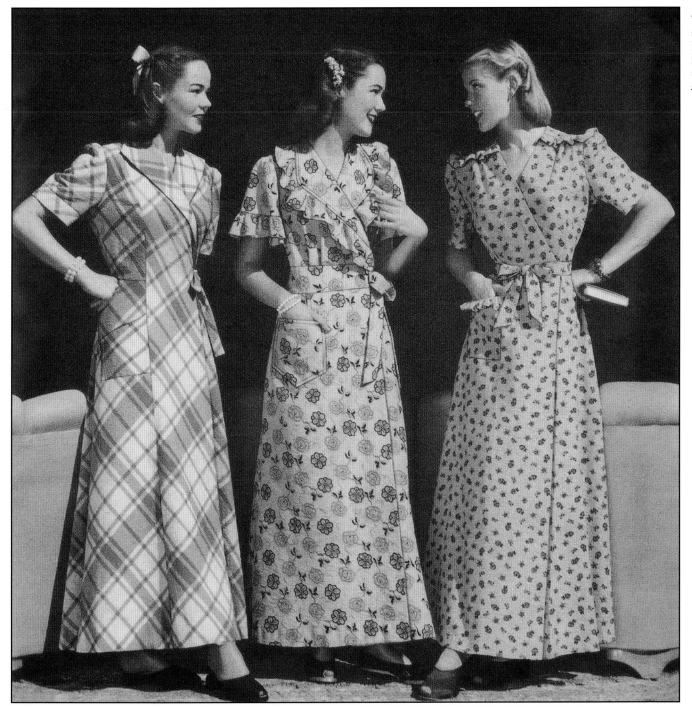

The smartest seersucker housecoats in slim styles with becoming necklines, all washable. Pastel plaid princess style, flower print with frills, or gay-printed extended shoulder style, in soft spring pastels. $5.29 each. [$5-10] *Spring/summer 1947*

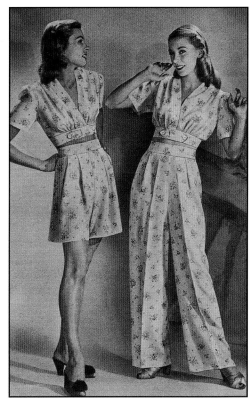

Shortie or Longie styles are cool, comfortable, and colorful. You can switch 'em, mix 'em, or match 'em. In attractive floral prints, on tearose or light blue grounds. $3-5. [$5-10] *Spring/summer 1947*

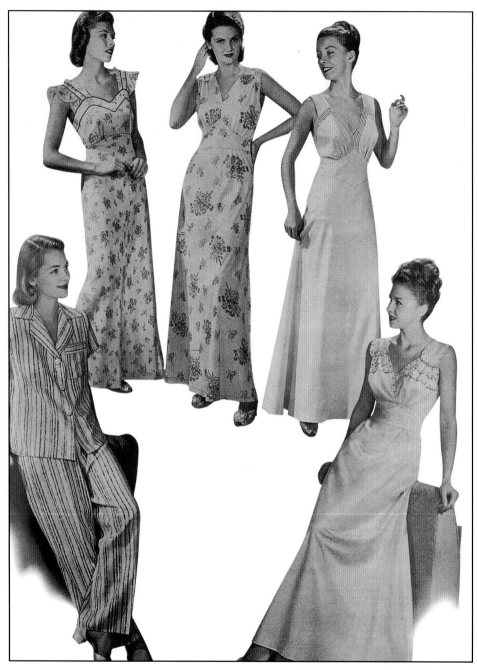

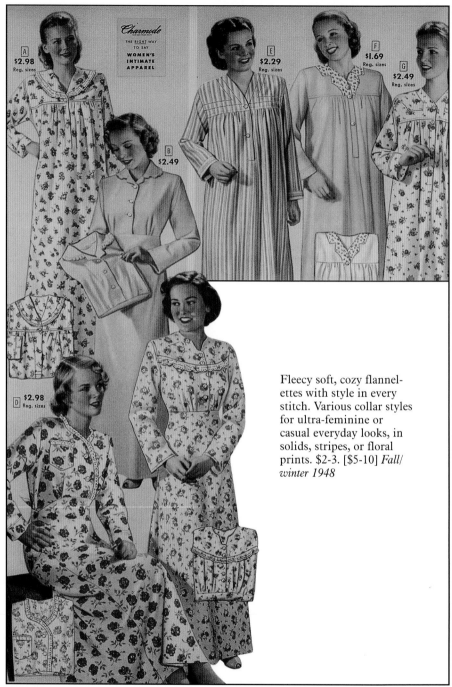

A $2.98 Reg. sizes

E $2.29 Reg. sizes

F $1.69 Reg. sizes

G $2.49 Reg. sizes

B $2.49

D $2.98 Reg. sizes

Fleecy soft, cozy flannel-ettes with style in every stitch. Various collar styles for ultra-feminine or casual everyday looks, in solids, stripes, or floral prints. $2-3. [$5-10] *Fall/winter 1948*

Charmode gowns and pajamas, pretty and practical. Breeze-cool and "fresh as spring." Rayon crepe, tricot knit rayon, and cotton voile fabrics, softest and most comfortable, in pale pink, pale blue, pale yellow, tearose, or assorted stripes and flower prints. $2-4. [$5-10] *Spring/summer 1947*

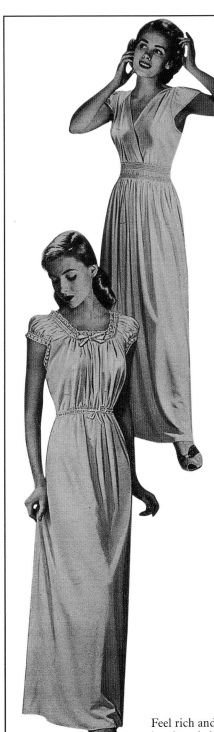

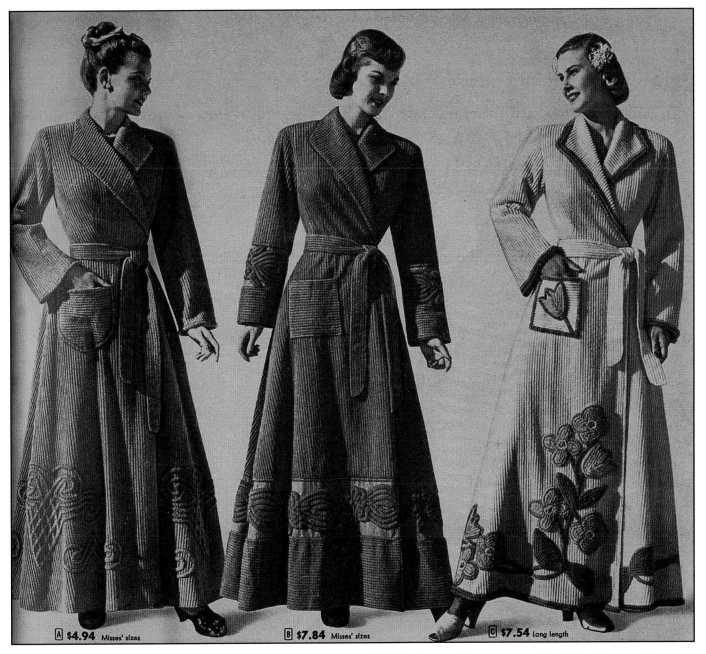

Pin point chenille Kerrybrooke robes are soft as velvet. All-around scroll design in aqua blue, rose, or medium blue. Flower and garland border on sleeves and skirt with double shawl collar, in rose, aqua blue, or medium blue. Multicolor floral print with smart double shawl collar, snow white with thickly tufted flowers in bright pastels. $5-9. [$15-20] *Fall/winter 1948*

Feel rich and petal-soft in these dainty knit rayon gowns. Run and wrinkle-resistant, hand-washable. Gracefully tailored with gathered bust sections, straight skirts and waist-hugging midriffs, in blue, tearose, or floral prints. $2-4. [$5-10] *Fall/winter 1948*

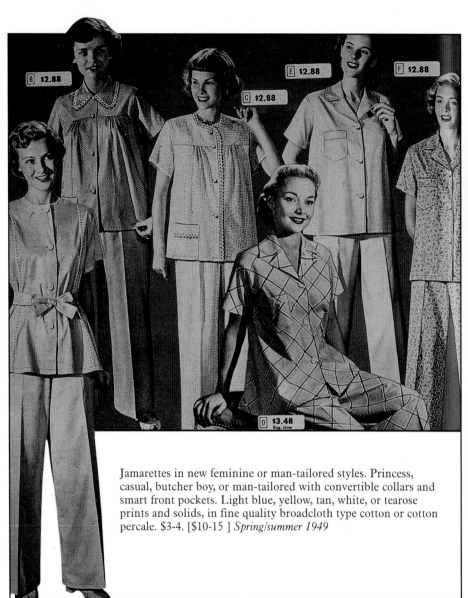

Jamarettes in new feminine or man-tailored styles. Princess, casual, butcher boy, or man-tailored with convertible collars and smart front pockets. Light blue, yellow, tan, white, or tearose prints and solids, in fine quality broadcloth type cotton or cotton percale. $3-4. [$10-15] *Spring/summer 1949*

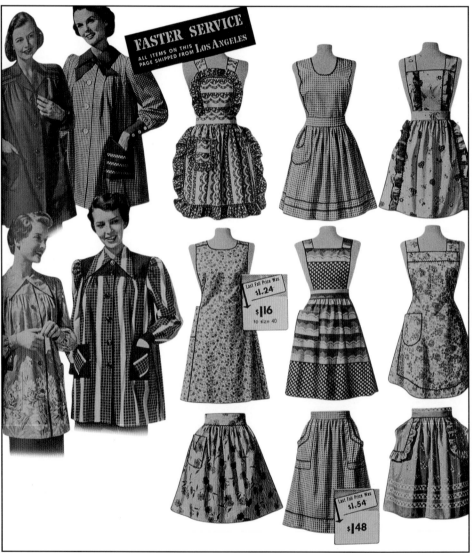

Cotton housecoats and smocks are grand to work in and generously cut for comfort. Great for the woman who works around the house. Ruffled, scalloped, polka-dotted, or pleated, these are made to last. In bright colors and assorted florals and prints. $1-2. [$5-10] *Spring/summer 1949*

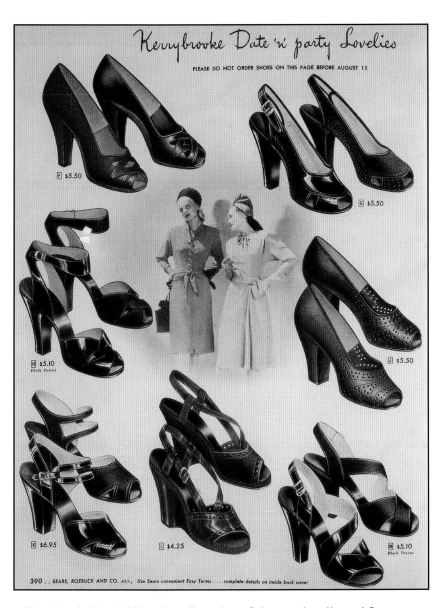

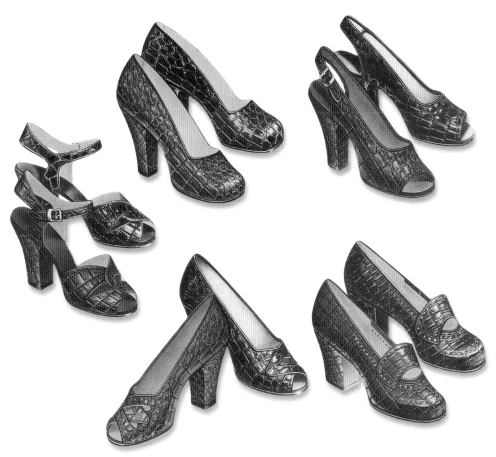

Alligator-grained calfskins are simple and smart. Fashion twist sandal, sling pump, and D'Orsay line styles, in handsome russet brown or black. $5-7. [$10-20] *Fall/winter 1946-1947*

Kerrybrooke Date 'n' Party Lovelies, wisps of glamour that slim and flatter your foot. Pumps and sandals in black patent, brown calf, and black suede or leather. $5-7. [$10-20] *Fall/winter 1946-1947*

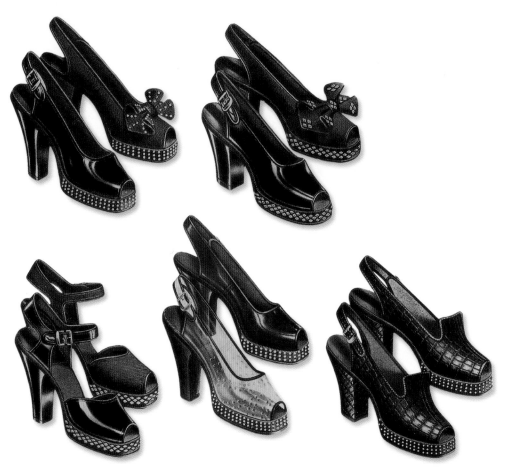

Nailhead-studded platforms by Kerrybrooke. Dramatic charm for gay evenings ahead, in black plastic or cotton gabardine. Beautiful cherry coke (brownish-red shiny plastic) or transparent vinyl sandal styles with red, green, or gold color nailheads. Easy-flex California-type construction. $5-6. [$10-20] *Fall/winter 1946-1947*

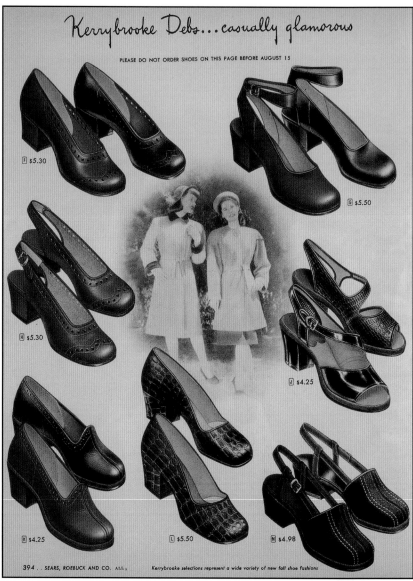

Perky, peppy fashion-model smartness with smooth Kerrybrooke fit and quality, low heels for high fashion! Baby doll toe, Shanksmare flats, and swing strap sandals, with open or closed backs, in brown and black leather or suede. $4-6. [$10-20] *Fall/winter 1946-1947*

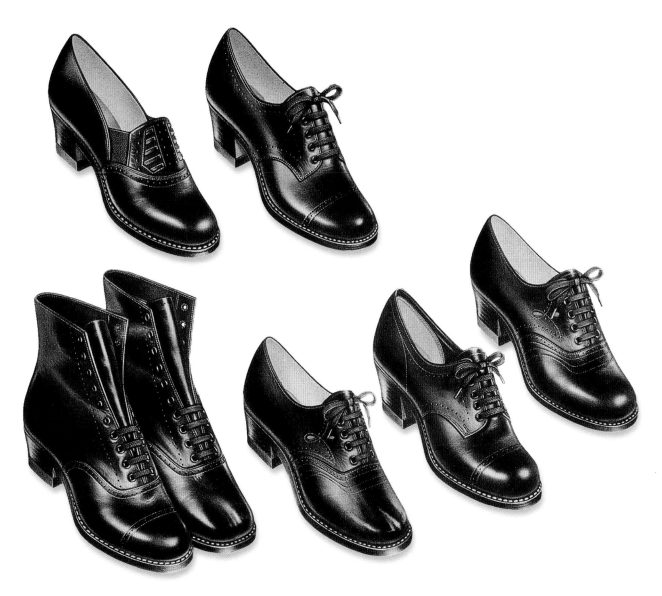

Comfort shoes to protect your feet from the jolts and jars of hard pavement. Offering all-day comfort, oxfords with flexible leather soles offer great support and soft or hard toe styles. In black leather or kidskin. $3-4. [$5-10] *Fall/winter 1946-1947*

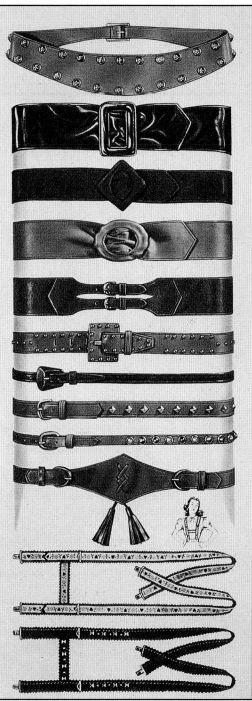

Waistline interest is important…beautiful belts for every occasion, richly studded or artfully plain. Patent-like plastic, capeskin, cowhide, and suede. $1-4. [$10-20] *Fall/winter 1946-1947*

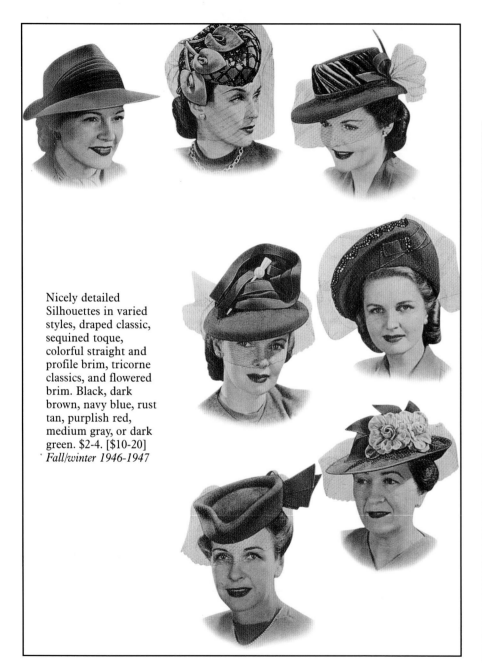

Nicely detailed Silhouettes in varied styles, draped classic, sequined toque, colorful straight and profile brim, tricorne classics, and flowered brim. Black, dark brown, navy blue, rust tan, purplish red, medium gray, or dark green. $2-4. [$10-20] *Fall/winter 1946-1947*

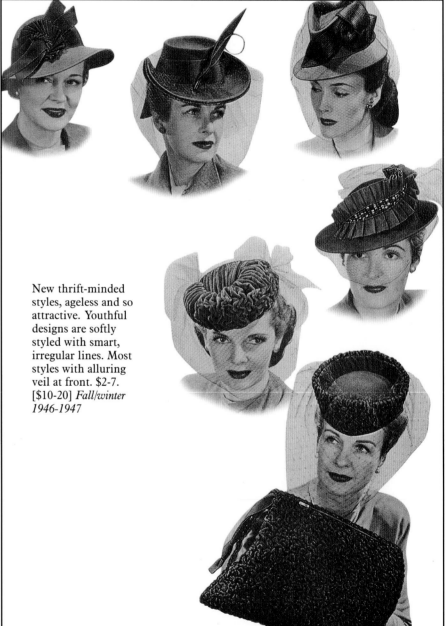

New thrift-minded styles, ageless and so attractive. Youthful designs are softly styled with smart, irregular lines. Most styles with alluring veil at front. $2-7. [$10-20] *Fall/winter 1946-1947*

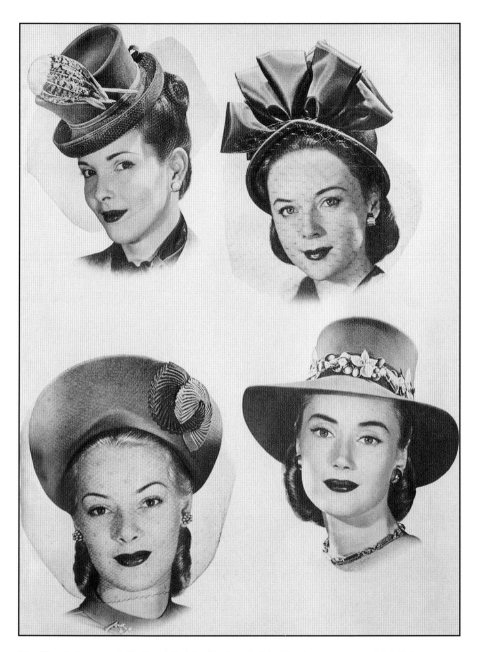

Postilion brim, carefully hand finished in lovely felt. Feather ornament highlights. Peaked front, lavish loops of matching rayon taffeta. Globe Breton, dramatic wool felt. Swagger brim, with casual seashell and glitter trim. $4-10. [$10-20] *Fall/winter 1946-1947*

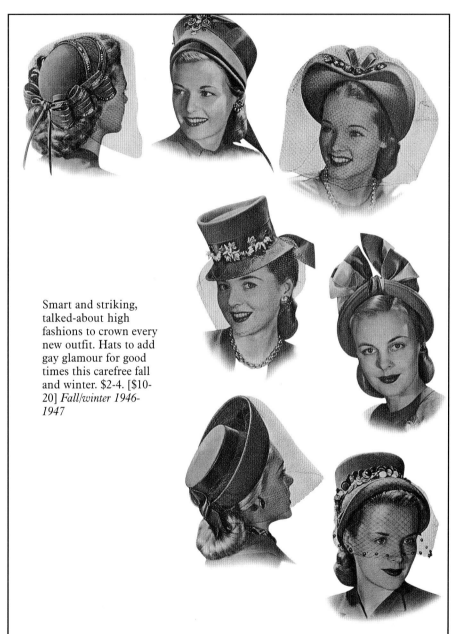

Smart and striking, talked-about high fashions to crown every new outfit. Hats to add gay glamour for good times this carefree fall and winter. $2-4. [$10-20] *Fall/winter 1946-1947*

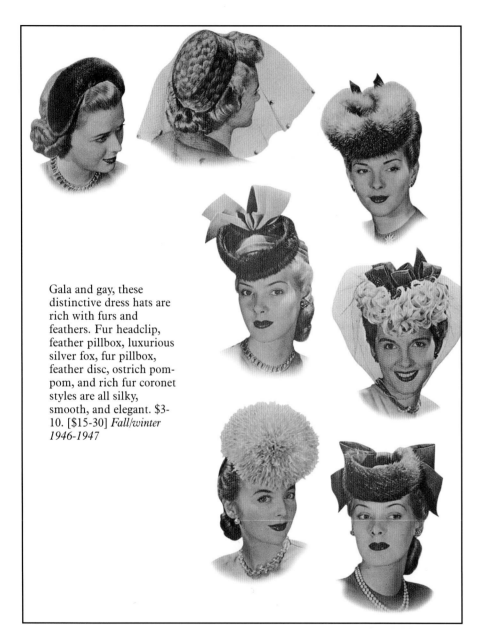

Gala and gay, these distinctive dress hats are rich with furs and feathers. Fur headclip, feather pillbox, luxurious silver fox, fur pillbox, feather disc, ostrich pom-pom, and rich fur coronet styles are all silky, smooth, and elegant. $3-10. [$15-30] *Fall/winter 1946-1947*

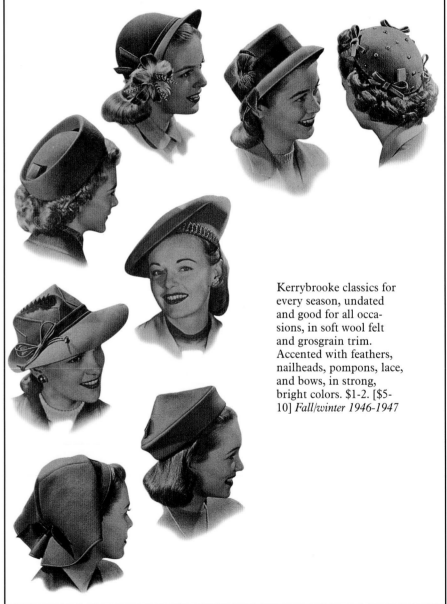

Kerrybrooke classics for every season, undated and good for all occasions, in soft wool felt and grosgrain trim. Accented with feathers, nailheads, pompons, lace, and bows, in strong, bright colors. $1-2. [$5-10] *Fall/winter 1946-1947*

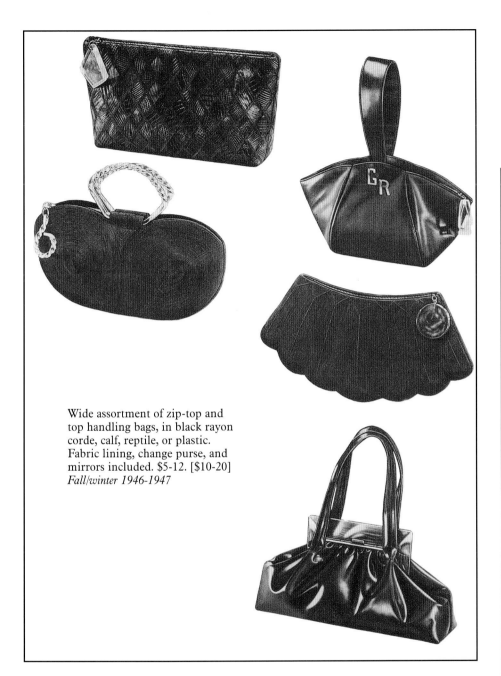

Wide assortment of zip-top and top handling bags, in black rayon corde, calf, reptile, or plastic. Fabric lining, change purse, and mirrors included. $5-12. [$10-20] *Fall/winter 1946-1947*

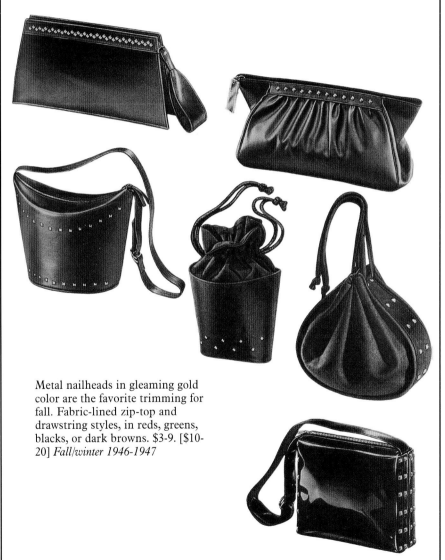

Metal nailheads in gleaming gold color are the favorite trimming for fall. Fabric-lined zip-top and drawstring styles, in reds, greens, blacks, or dark browns. $3-9. [$10-20] *Fall/winter 1946-1947*

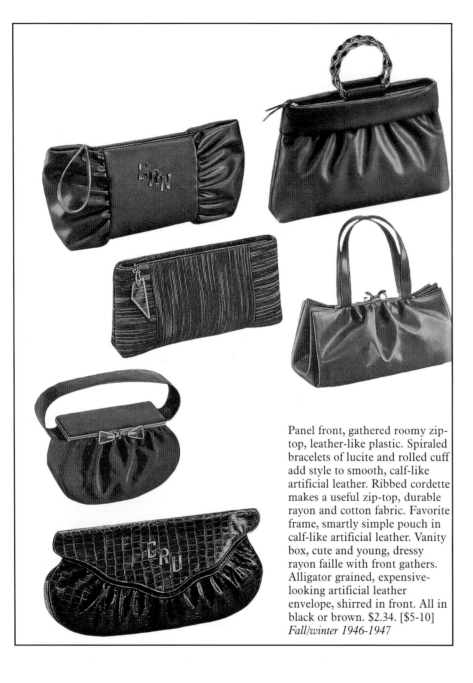

Panel front, gathered roomy zip-top, leather-like plastic. Spiraled bracelets of lucite and rolled cuff add style to smooth, calf-like artificial leather. Ribbed cordette makes a useful zip-top, durable rayon and cotton fabric. Favorite frame, smartly simple pouch in calf-like artificial leather. Vanity box, cute and young, dressy rayon faille with front gathers. Alligator grained, expensive-looking artificial leather envelope, shirred in front. All in black or brown. $2.34. [$5-10] *Fall/winter 1946-1947*

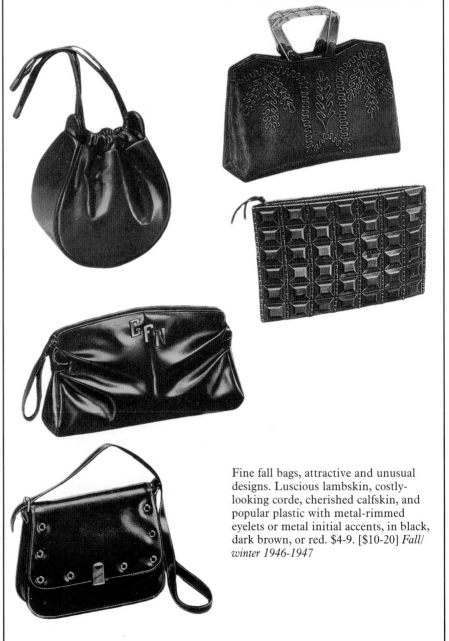

Fine fall bags, attractive and unusual designs. Luscious lambskin, costly-looking corde, cherished calfskin, and popular plastic with metal-rimmed eyelets or metal initial accents, in black, dark brown, or red. $4-9. [$10-20] *Fall/winter 1946-1947*

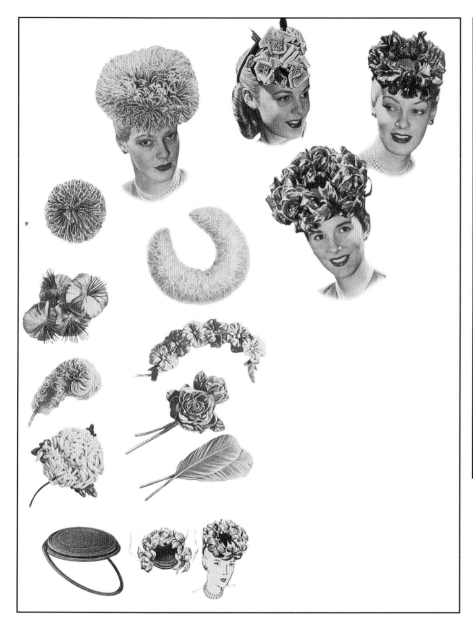

Feathers or flowers look extravagant, use them to trim a disc for smart effect. For a more elegant look, ostrich sprays or pom-poms add height and grace. Crossed quills, roses, chrysanthemums, and marabous look great on a date or at an important engagement with your husband. $1-4. [$5-7] *Fall/winter 1946-1947*

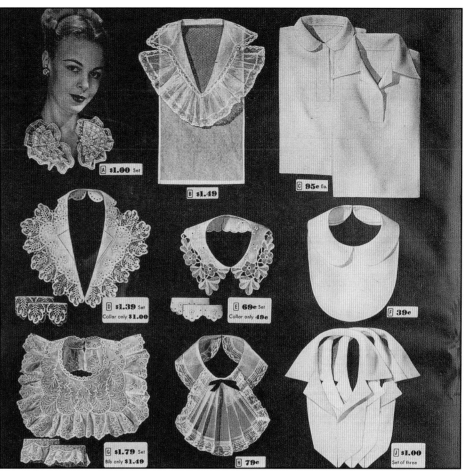

Change your dresses and suits with hand-washable neckwear. Crisp cotton or firm rayon, in various neckline styles. Great for adding some flavor to a plain wardrobe or emphasizing your fabulously feminine outfits, with cuff and pocket clip-ons, too. 50¢-$1. [$3-5] *Spring/summer 1947*

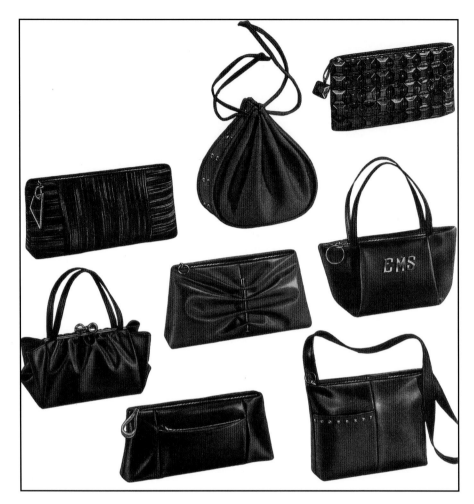

Leather-like plastics, soft fabrics, plastic cubes, and fashionable felt. Great new drawstring and zip-top styles for summer, some with nailhead accents. $2.34. [$10-15] *Spring/summer 1947*

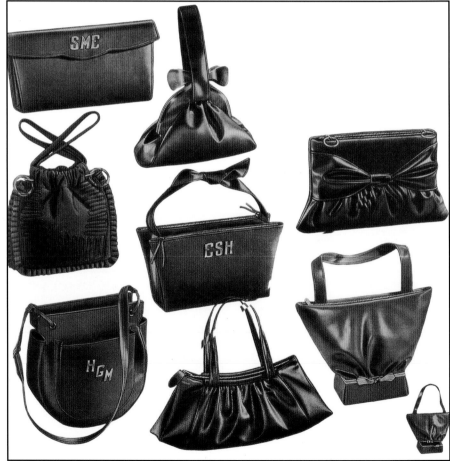

Five-section envelope, dressmaker pouch, postman style, drawstring with lively embroidery, side-pocket carryall, or vanity bag with bottom-snapping cosmetic container. New novelties in fashion, perfect to dress up and accent any outfit. $3.49. [$10-15] *Spring/summer 1947*

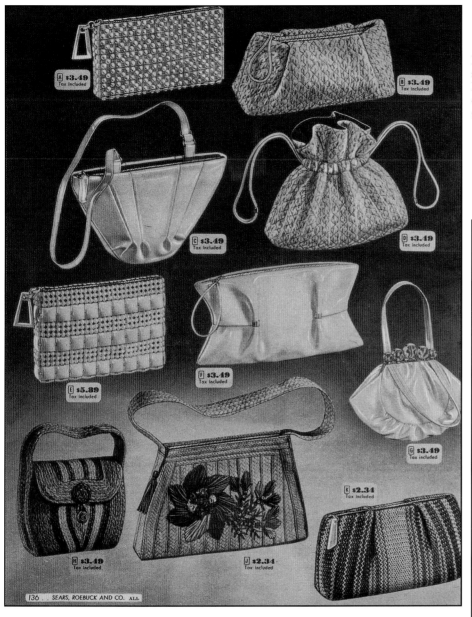

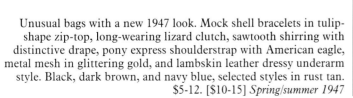

Bright white or vivid color for your warm weather bags. Dramatic new shapes heighten the effect of the smart textures and clever trimmings. Bubble cubes, beads, colorful quilting, or sparkling shoulderstrap in cool white patent-like plastic, summery straw, or rainbow stripe sisals, shoulder bags, and clutches. $2-6. [$10-15] *Spring/summer 1947*

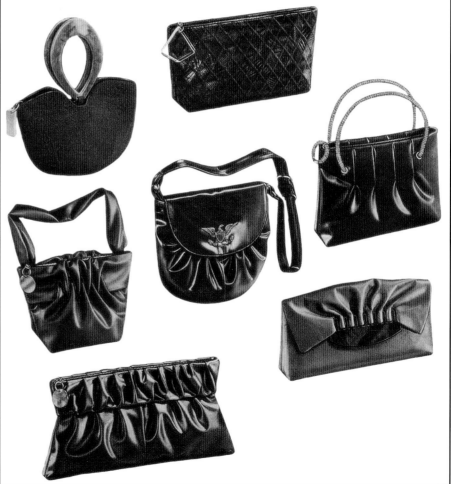

Unusual bags with a new 1947 look. Mock shell bracelets in tulip-shape zip-top, long-wearing lizard clutch, sawtooth shirring with distinctive drape, pony express shoulderstrap with American eagle, metal mesh in glittering gold, and lambskin leather dressy underarm style. Black, dark brown, and navy blue, selected styles in rust tan. $5-12. [$10-15] *Spring/summer 1947*

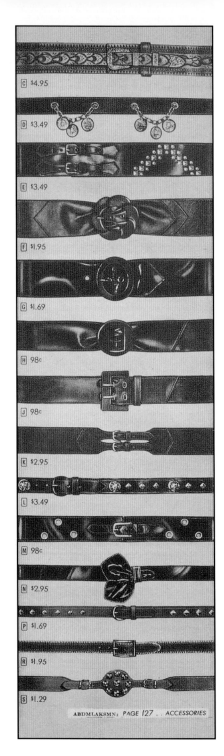

One of these eye-catching belts makes the simplest outfit more important. Capeskin leather, calf-like and patent-like plastic, or cowhide. $1-4. [$5-10] *Spring/summer 1947*

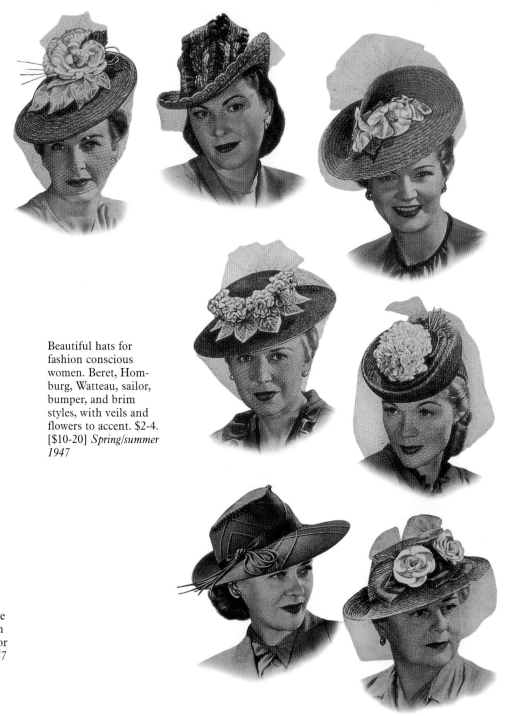

Beautiful hats for fashion conscious women. Beret, Homburg, Watteau, sailor, bumper, and brim styles, with veils and flowers to accent. $2-4. [$10-20] *Spring/summer 1947*

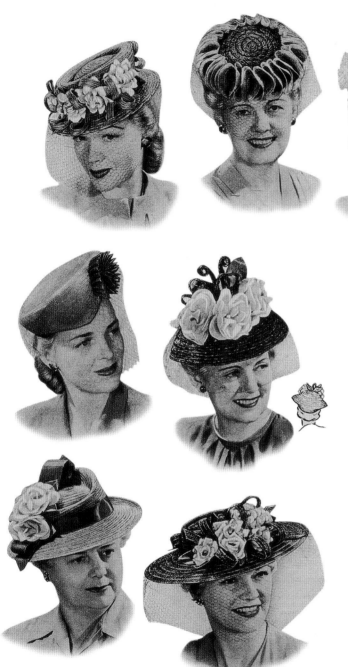

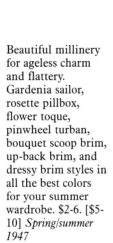

Beautiful millinery for ageless charm and flattery. Gardenia sailor, rosette pillbox, flower toque, pinwheel turban, bouquet scoop brim, up-back brim, and dressy brim styles in all the best colors for your summer wardrobe. $2-6. [$5-10] *Spring/summer 1947*

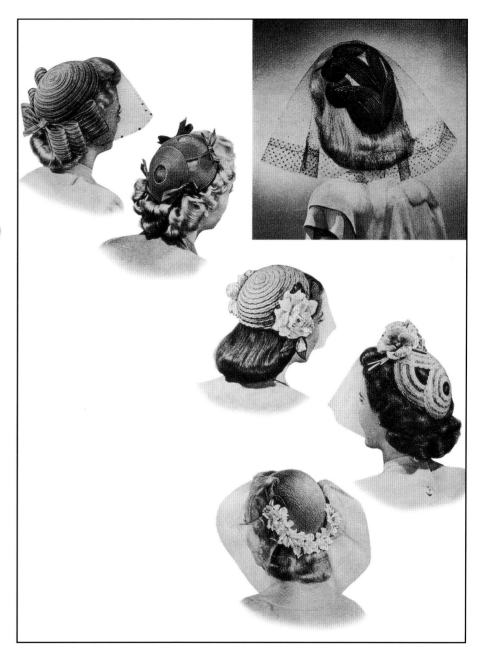

Calots are young and carefree, correct with every costume. Bows and flowers fabulously flatter. Red, navy, black, white, rose, golden tan, or medium blue. $2-3. [$5-10] *Spring/summer 1947*

61

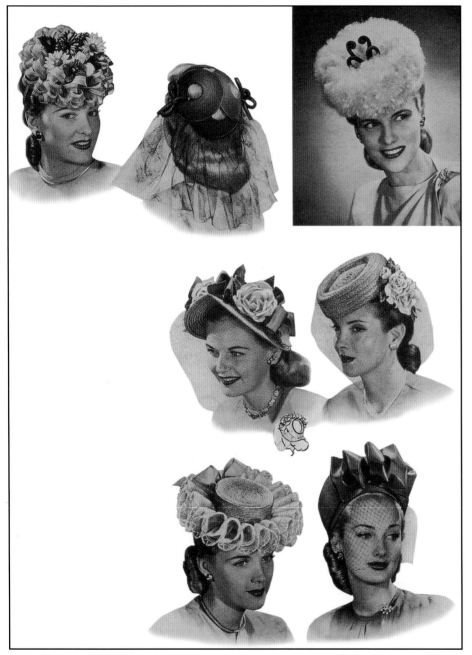

Sophisticated and wearable, frankly feminine and flattering, field flower discs, three-ring calots, marabou powder puff, pillboxes, and turbans are good dress-up strategies. $2-4. [$10-15] *Spring/summer 1947*

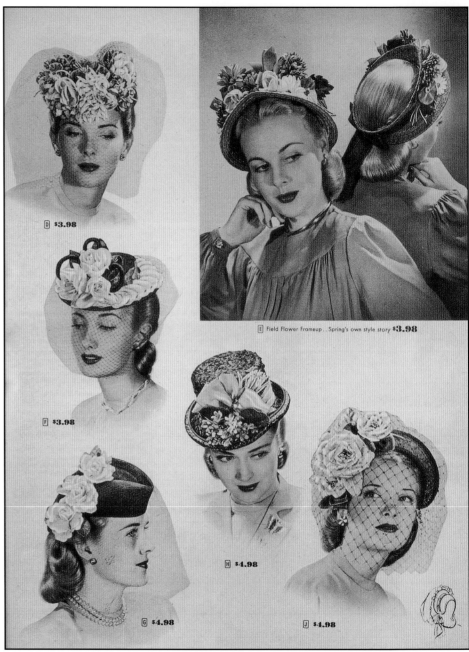

D $3.98

E Field Flower Frameup...Spring's own style story $3.98

F $3.98

G $4.98

H $4.98

J $4.98

Head-turning hats…the exclamation point of your outfit. Each is a whole new world of fashion and a wealth of feminine flattery in flowers and veils. $4-5. [$5-10] *Spring/summer 1947*

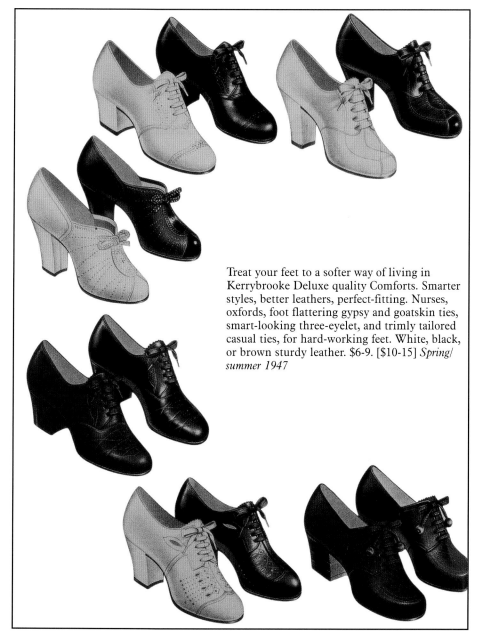

Treat your feet to a softer way of living in Kerrybrooke Deluxe quality Comforts. Smarter styles, better leathers, perfect-fitting. Nurses, oxfords, foot flattering gypsy and goatskin ties, smart-looking three-eyelet, and trimly tailored casual ties, for hard-working feet. White, black, or brown sturdy leather. $6-9. [$10-15] *Spring/ summer 1947*

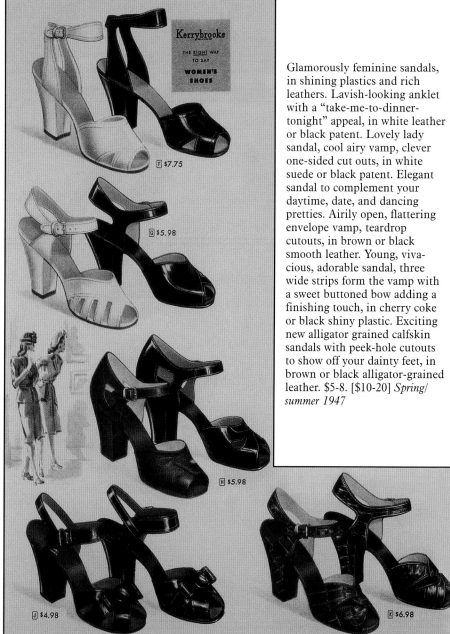

Glamorously feminine sandals, in shining plastics and rich leathers. Lavish-looking anklet with a "take-me-to-dinner-tonight" appeal, in white leather or black patent. Lovely lady sandal, cool airy vamp, clever one-sided cut outs, in white suede or black patent. Elegant sandal to complement your daytime, date, and dancing pretties. Airily open, flattering envelope vamp, teardrop cutouts, in brown or black smooth leather. Young, vivacious, adorable sandal, three wide strips form the vamp with a sweet buttoned bow adding a finishing touch, in cherry coke or black shiny plastic. Exciting new alligator grained calfskin sandals with peek-hole cutouts to show off your dainty feet, in brown or black alligator-grained leather. $5-8. [$10-20] *Spring/ summer 1947*

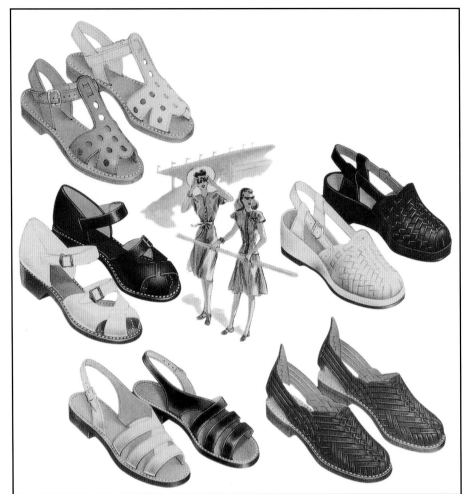

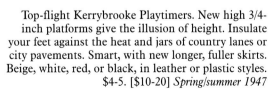

Carefree barefoot sandal flatties are yours for a fun-filled summer. Open, airy, refreshingly young. Grand for pitter-pattering around the house, for gardening, marketing, or sports. Foot-caressing leather, in beige, white, brown, or black. $2-5. [$10-20] *Spring/summer 1947*

Top-flight Kerrybrooke Playtimers. New high 3/4-inch platforms give the illusion of height. Insulate your feet against the heat and jars of country lanes or city pavements. Smart, with new longer, fuller skirts. Beige, white, red, or black, in leather or plastic styles. $4-5. [$10-20] *Spring/summer 1947*

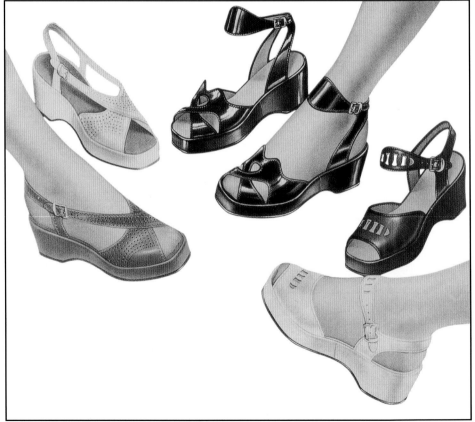

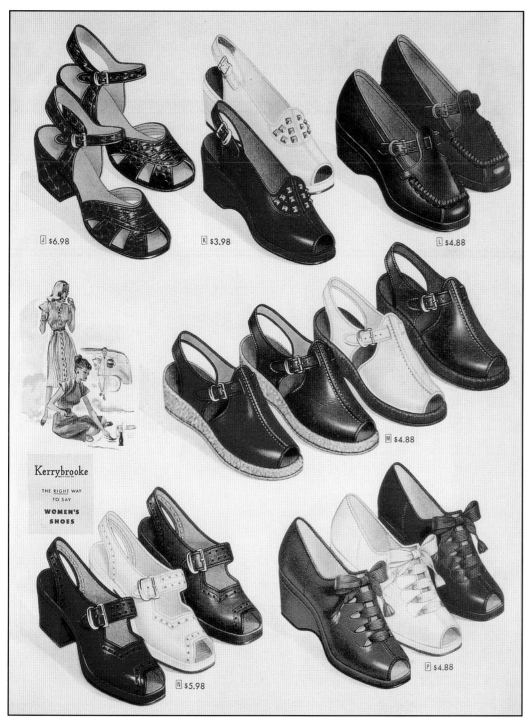

Kerrybrooke

THE RIGHT WAY
TO SAY
WOMEN'S SHOES

J $6.98

K $3.98

L $4.88

M $4.88

N $5.98

P $4.88

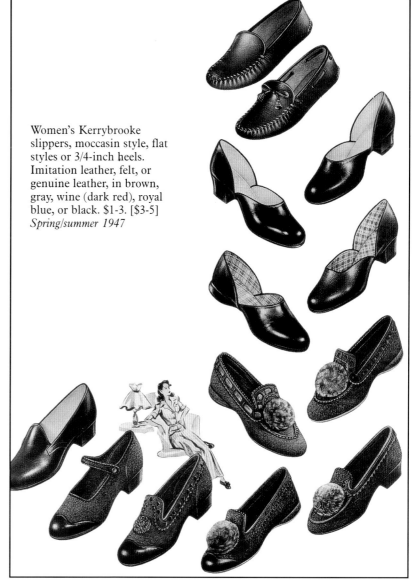

Women's Kerrybrooke slippers, moccasin style, flat styles or 3/4-inch heels. Imitation leather, felt, or genuine leather, in brown, gray, wine (dark red), royal blue, or black. $1-3. [$3-5] *Spring/summer 1947*

Fun-in-the-Sun Kerrybrookes are so light, so cool, and so foot-flattering. Butter-soft leathers and flower-fresh colors come in lots of fun styles. Alligator-grained calfskins, nailhead-studded peaked vamp shanksmares, sturdy T-strap soft toe sandals, two exciting new sandal styles, and gay-hearted ties. Lots of bright, summer colors. $4-7. [$10-20] *Spring/summer 1947*

65

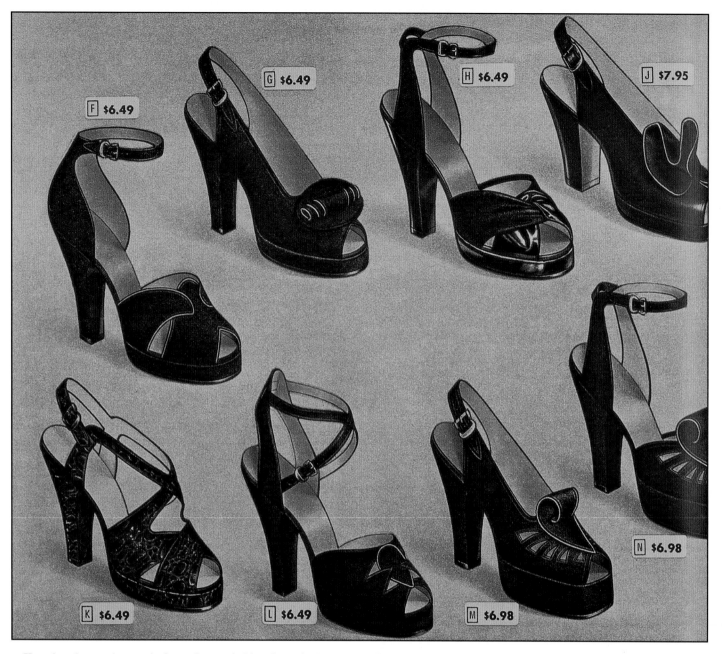

F $6.49   G $6.49   H $6.49   J $7.95

K $6.49   L $6.49   M $6.98   N $6.98

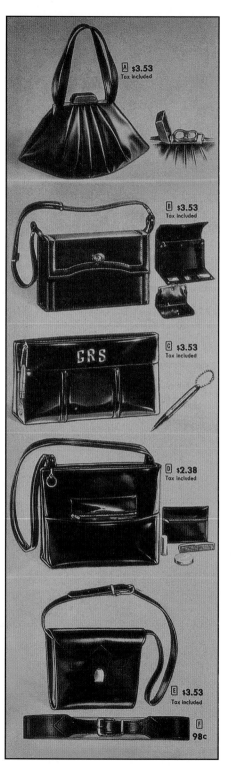

A $3.53 Tax included

B $3.53 Tax included

C $3.53 Tax included

D $2.38 Tax included

E $3.53 Tax included

F 98c

Kerrybrooke nominates platforms for top fashion favor, for beauty, and for comfort. Three inch-or-more heels give you a gay lift and a minimizing look. Exquisite sandals and sling pumps in smooth leather, patent, or jungle alligator-grained styles. $6-8. [$10-20] *Fall/winter 1948*

New bags full of tricks! Fitted with a variety of useful accessories, handy to carry. Coin holder bag, ballpoint pen bag, makeup kit, go-everywhere shoulder bag styles, in black, red, or brown. $2-4. [$10-15] *Fall/winter 1948*

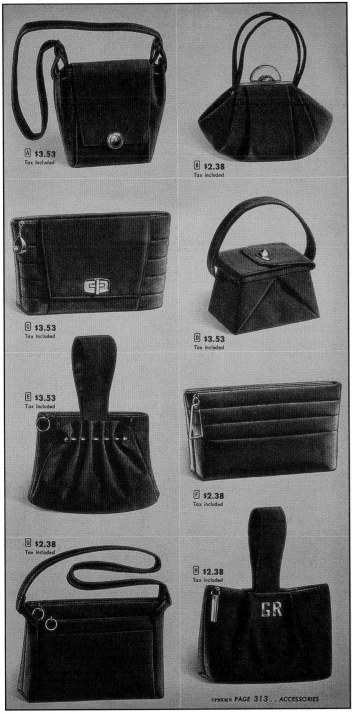

A $3.53
Tax Included

B $2.38
Tax Included

C $3.53
Tax Included

D $3.53
Tax Included

E $3.53
Tax Included

F $2.38
Tax Included

G $2.38
Tax Included

H $2.38
Tax Included

GR

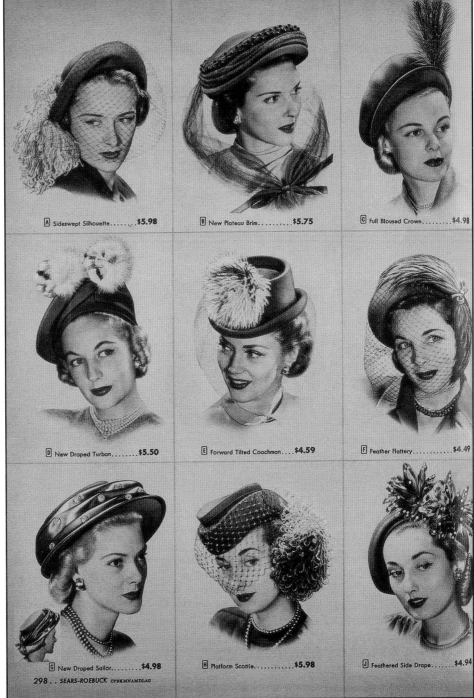

A Sideswept Silhouette.........$5.98

B New Plateau Brim.........$5.75

C Full Bloused Crown.........$4.98

D New Draped Turban.........$5.50

E Forward Tilted Coachman....$4.59

F Feather Flattery.........$4.49

G New Draped Sailor.........$4.98

H Platform Scottie.........$5.98

J Feathered Side Drape.......$4.94

LEFT Suede-like plastics boast the rich elegance and soft texture of suede. They wear well and look stunning with your clothes. Shoulder swingers, top handlers, and underarm clutches. Selected styles in black, wine red, brown, and dark green. $2-4. [$10-15] *Fall/winter 1948*

RIGHT · Hats were never so wonderful, so imaginative, so really essential to the success of your longer, more feminine fashions. Winter browns, beiges, whites, grays, and blacks. $4-6. [$10-15] *Fall/winter 1948*

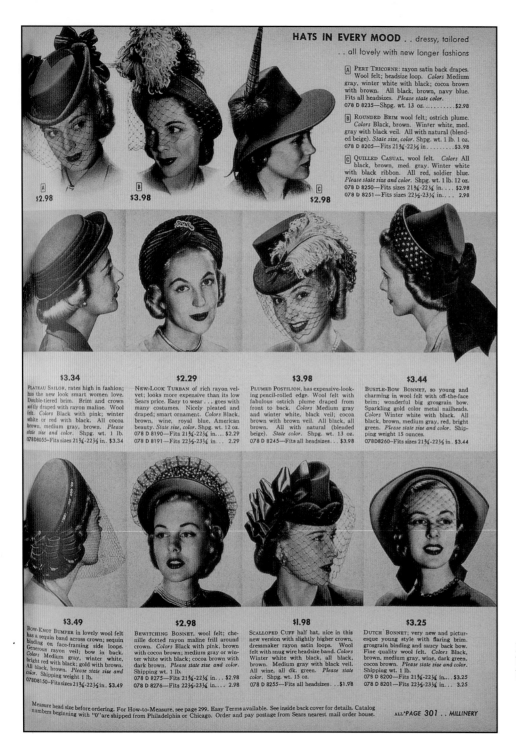

HATS IN EVERY MOOD .. dressy, tailored
.. all lovely with new longer fashions

A PERT TRICORNE: rayon satin back drapes. Wool felt; headsize loop. *Colors* Medium gray, winter white with black; cocoa brown with brown. All black, brown, navy blue. Fits all headsizes. *Please state color.*
078 D 8235—Shpg. wt. 13 oz. $2.98

B ROUNDED BRIM wool felt; ostrich plume. *Colors* Black, brown. Winter white, med. gray with black veil. All with natural (blended beige). *State size, color.* Shpg. wt. 1 lb. 1 oz.
078 D 8205—Fits 21¾-22½ in. $3.98

C QUILLED CASUAL, wool felt. *Colors* All black, brown, med. gray. Winter white with black ribbon. All red, soldier blue. *Please state size and color.* Shpg. wt. 12 oz.
078 D 8250—Fits sizes 21¾-22½ in. . . . $2.98
078 D 8251—Fits sizes 22½-23¼ in. . . . 2.98

$2.98 **$3.98** **$2.98**

$3.34
PLATEAU SAILOR, rates high in fashion; has the new look smart women love. Double-tiered brim. Brim and crown softly draped with rayon maline. Wool felt. *Colors* Black with pink; winter white or red with black. All cocoa brown, medium gray, brown. *Please state size and color.*
078D8055-Fits sizes 21¾-22½ in. $3.34

$2.29
NEW-LOOK TURBAN of rich rayon velvet; looks more expensive than its low Sears price. Easy to wear . . . goes with many costumes. Nicely pleated and draped; smart ornament. *Colors* Black, brown, wine, royal blue, American beauty. *State size, color.* Shpg. wt. 12 oz.
078 D 8190—Fits 21¾-22½ in. . . $2.29
078 D 8191—Fits 22½-23¼ in. . . 2.29

$3.98
PLUMED POSTILION, has expensive-looking pencil-rolled edge. Wool felt with fabulous ostrich plume draped from front to back. *Colors* Medium gray and winter white, black veil; cocoa brown with brown veil. All black, all brown. All with natural (blended beige). *State color.* Shpg. wt. 13 oz.
078 D 8245—Fits all headsizes . . . $3.98

$3.44
BUSTLE-BOW BONNET, so young and charming in wool felt with off-the-face brim; wonderful big grosgrain bow. Sparkling gold color metal nailheads. *Colors* Winter white with black, black brown, medium gray, red, bright green. *Please state size and color.* Shipping weight 15 ounces.
078D8260—Fits sizes 21¾-22½ in. $3.44

$3.49
BOW-KNOT BUMPER in lovely wool felt has a sequin band across crown; sequin binding on face-framing side loops. Generous rayon veil; bow in back. *Colors* Medium gray, winter white, bright red with black; gold with brown. All black, brown. *Please state size and color.* Shipping weight 1 lb.
078D8150-Fits sizes 21¾-22½ in. $3.49

$2.98
BEWITCHING BONNET, wool felt; chenille dotted rayon maline frill around crown. *Colors* Black with pink, brown with cocoa brown; medium gray or winter white with black; cocoa brown with dark brown. *Please state size and color.* Shipping wt. 1 lb.
078 D 8275—Fits sizes 21¾-22½ in. . . $2.98
078 D 8276—Fits sizes 22½-23¼ in. . . . 2.98

$1.98
SCALLOPED CUFF half hat, nice in this new version with slightly higher crown, dressmaker rayon satin loops. Wool felt with snug wire headsize band. *Colors* Winter white with black, all black, brown. Medium gray with black veil. All wine, all dk. green. *Please state color.* Shpg. wt. 15 oz.
078 D 8255—Fits all headsizes . . . $1.98

$3.25
DUTCH BONNET; very new and picturesque young style with flaring brim. grosgrain binding and saucy back bow. Fine quality wool felt. *Colors* Black, brown, medium gray, wine, dark green, cocoa brown. *Please state size and color.* Shipping wt. 1 lb.
078 D 8200—Fits 21¾-22½ in. . . . $3.25
078 D 8201—Fits 22½-23¼ in. . . . 3.25

Measure head size before ordering. For How-to-Measure, see page 299. Easy Terms available. See inside back cover for details. Catalog numbers beginning with "0" are shipped from Philadelphia or Chicago. Order and pay postage from Sears nearest mail order house.

ALL°PAGE 301 . . MILLINERY

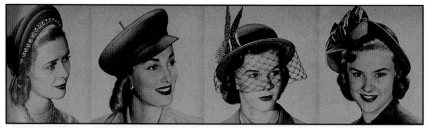

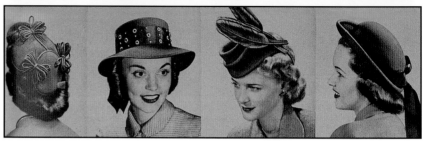

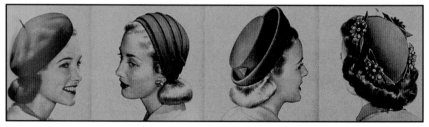

Kerrybrooke classics…choose from these smart little hat-hits, in popular colors and tailored or dressy styles. Bloused crown visor cap, dashing sailor, demure bonnet, dip-brim casual, Scottie half-hat, saucy derby, imported Basque beret, slick little helmet, popular Breton, or bow-and-flower calot. $2. [$10-15] *Fall/winter 1948*

Hats in every mood. Dressy tailored, all lovely with new longer fashions. Rounded brim, quilled casual, new-look turban, plumed postilion, bustle-bow or bewitching bonnet, scalloped cuff half hat, or Dutch bonnet styles. $2-4. [$10-15] *Fall/winter 1948*

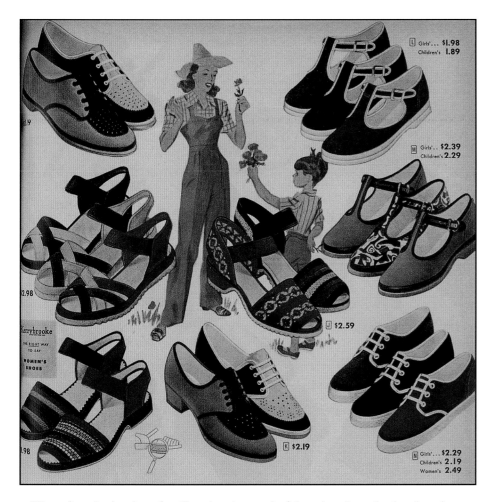

L Girls'... $1.98
Children's 1.89

M Girls'.. $2.39
Children's 2.29

J $2.59

K $2.19

N Girls'.. $2.29
Children's 2.19
Women's 2.49

2.98

Kerrybrooke
THE RIGHT WAY
TO SAY
WOMEN'S
SHOES

1.98

Women's and misses' carefree Kerrybrookes...colorful, cool, and sturdy play shoes in lightweight, washable cottons. Breeze along in airy comfort with multiple styles. Oxfords, barefoot sandal honeys, and feather-light sandals with striped vamps. Lovely in any setting. $2-3. [$10] *Spring/summer 1949*

Pick bright, colorful leather play shoes for sun-filled hours. Easy-comfort California-style platforms with wedge heels. Styles include smoothie ties, play-minded wedgies, leather ties, Haiti-inspired sandals, pool-cool bracelet sandals, and comfortable U-throated leather ties. $5. Raffia-weave shoulder bag, in red, natural tan, or black. $3. *Spring/summer 1949*

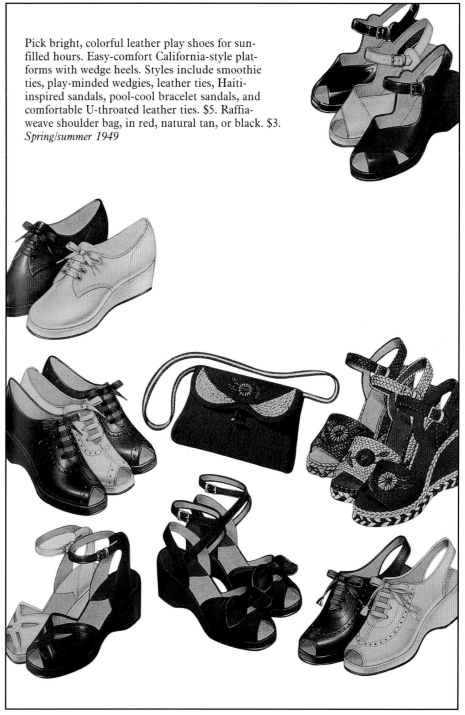

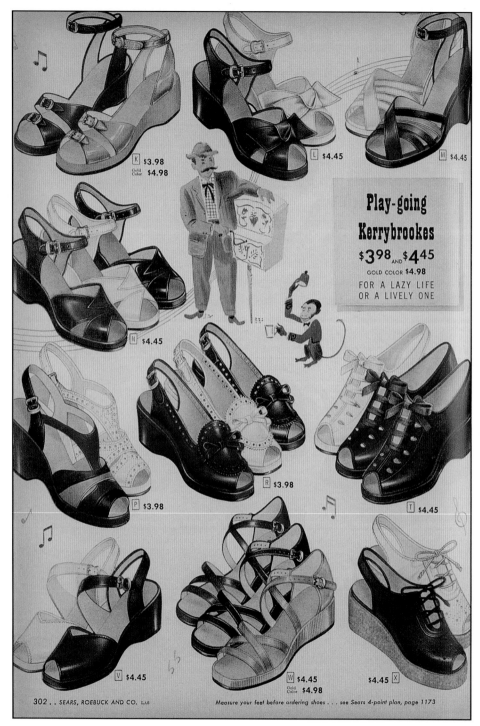

K $3.98
Gold Color $4.98

L $4.45

M $4.45

N $4.45

R $3.98

P $3.98

T $4.45

V $4.45

W $4.45
Gold Color $4.98

$4.45 X

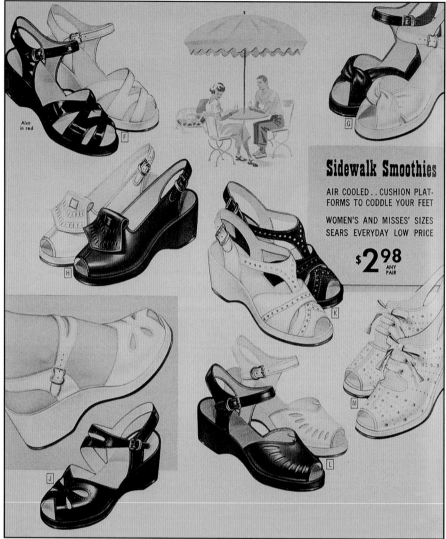

Also in red

F

G

H

J

K

L

M

Sidewalk Smoothies…air-cooled cushion platforms to coddle your feet. Leather sandals in lots of styles. Air-cooling shapely vamps, dainty straps, and sling-ons. With wedge heels and California platforms. In red, white, black, or brown. $3. [$10-15] *Spring/summer 1949*

Play-going Kerrybrooke recipes for a light-footed summer. Shoes made the softly cushioned, California way for a lazy life or a lively one. Smooth leathers and vibrant colors…cool as the dew-drenched flowers. $4-5. [$10-15] *Spring/summer 1949*

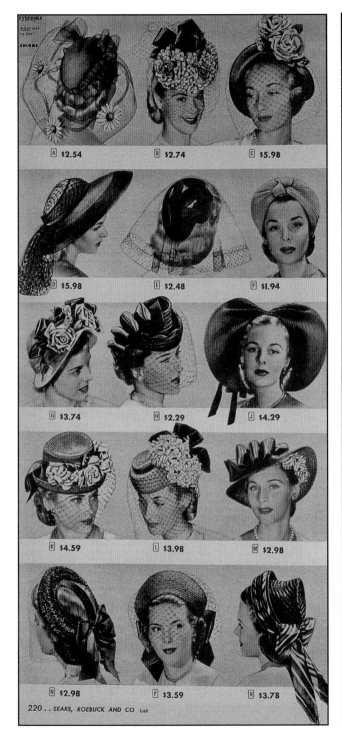

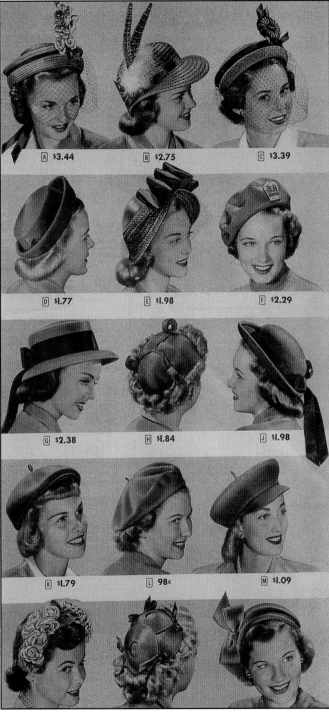

LEFT · Flattering hats in a rich variety of the season's loveliest styles, beauty and fashion for every type. Straw braid hats with luscious flowers, rayon veils, and taffeta ribbons in a variety of colors and styles. Choose from feather-light sisal straw, big sweep brim, glamour calot, turban, Homburg, fine straw braid Scotty, or off-the-face bonnet, among others. $2-5. [$10-15] *Spring/summer 1949*

RIGHT · Kerrybrooke hat-hits that make you look the prettiest. Beautiful Bretons, bonnets, berets, calots, caps, and derbies. In lots of colors, select styles with bows, feathers, flowers, and veils. $1-4. [$10-15] *Spring/summer 1949*

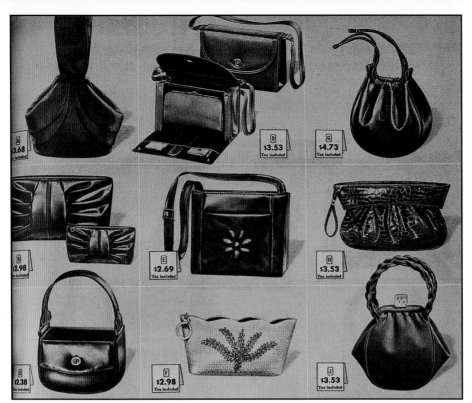

Kerrybrooke bags add elegance and beauty to any outfit. All your style and color needs. Faille, fitted shoulder, lambskin drawstring, two-in-one treat, flower-front, cuff-top underarm, box bag, gala and braided tophandle bags. $3-4. [$10-15] *Spring/summer 1949*

Patent-like plastic sparkling as spring in a variety of styles. You'll love their expensive-looking lines. They'll wear and wear…won't scuff, crack, or peel…can be wiped down easily. Enjoy all the styles. Outside pocket, busy women's delight, dainty panier-handled pouch, three-zipper underarm bag, buckled beauty, button bag, dramatic tophandle, underarm ziptop, and lovely lucite catch. In black or white. $2-4. [$10-15] *Spring/summer 1949*

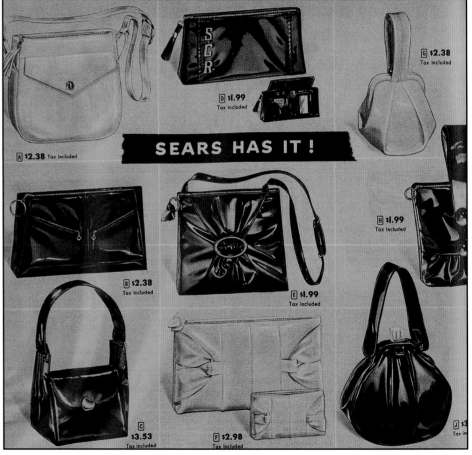

Dresses

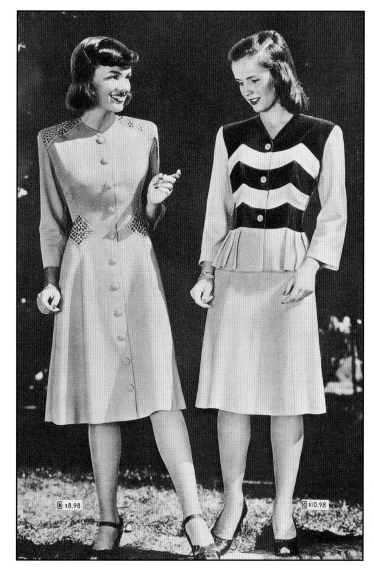

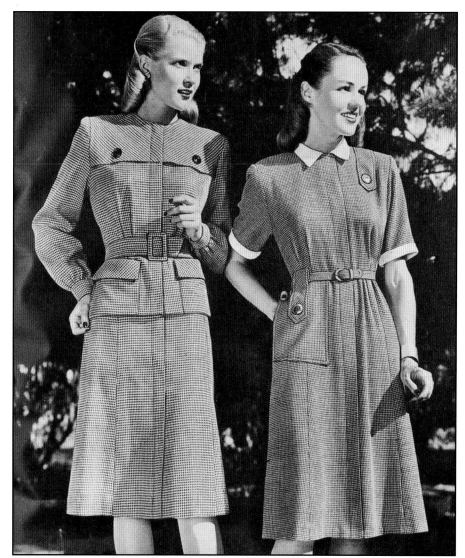

Neat, checked cotton dresses, heartbreakers with smart tabs and buttons…school, work, or date dresses. Tweed checked two-piece, woven-check cotton suiting in Basque suit style. Checked print cotton suiting with make-believe fly front, crisp white collar and cuffs. Both in black and white checks. $6, $4. [$10-20] *Fall/winter 1946-1947*

Juniors…perky new styles and vivid young colors that only you can wear. Princess silhouette style, shining nailheads sharpen shoulder yoke. Crease-resistant rayon gabardine, in light coral red or gold. Tempting two-piecer in 50% wool and 50% rayon, contrasting cotton velveteen insert bands, medium blue with dark brown, light coral with black, gold with dark brown, or aqua blue with black. $9-11. [$10-20] *Fall/winter 1946-1947*

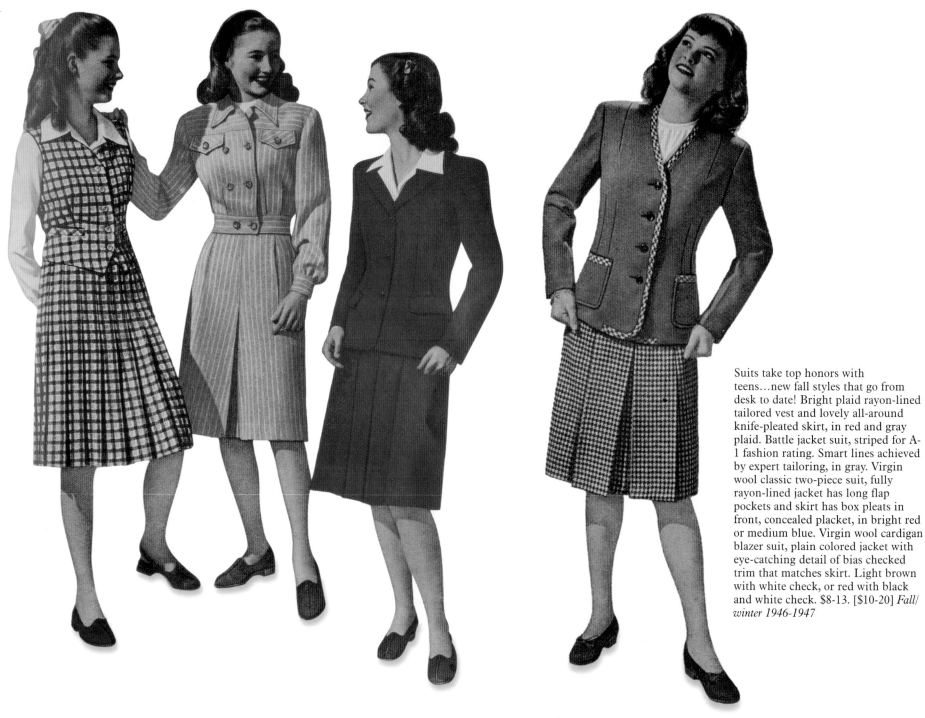

Suits take top honors with teens…new fall styles that go from desk to date! Bright plaid rayon-lined tailored vest and lovely all-around knife-pleated skirt, in red and gray plaid. Battle jacket suit, striped for A-1 fashion rating. Smart lines achieved by expert tailoring, in gray. Virgin wool classic two-piece suit, fully rayon-lined jacket has long flap pockets and skirt has box pleats in front, concealed placket, in bright red or medium blue. Virgin wool cardigan blazer suit, plain colored jacket with eye-catching detail of bias checked trim that matches skirt. Light brown with white check, or red with black and white check. $8-13. [$10-20] *Fall/winter 1946-1947*

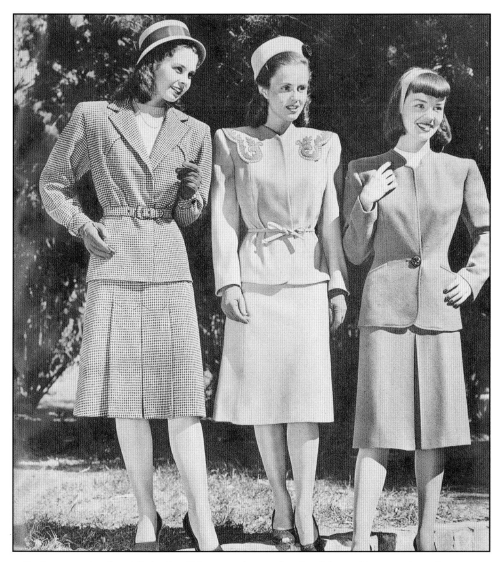

Juniors…you're the girls in the slick new suits…you're the girls working overtime. A shirtwaist suit in pure wool checks, wrist-tight cuffs on winged sleeves, black-and-white or brown-and-white check. Cardigan suit in dressy all wool crepe, contrasting scallop embroidery and string-tied middle, in gray, medium brown, medium green, or black. Notch-necked suit in lovely domestic Shetland-type wool. Figure-following rayon-lined jacket, in medium brown, medium blue, gold, or medium green. $13-17. [$10-20] *Fall/winter 1946-1947*

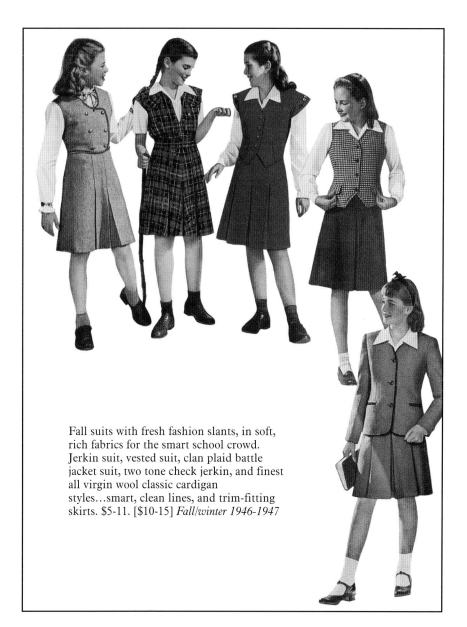

Fall suits with fresh fashion slants, in soft, rich fabrics for the smart school crowd. Jerkin suit, vested suit, clan plaid battle jacket suit, two tone check jerkin, and finest all virgin wool classic cardigan styles…smart, clean lines, and trim-fitting skirts. $5-11. [$10-15] *Fall/winter 1946-1947*

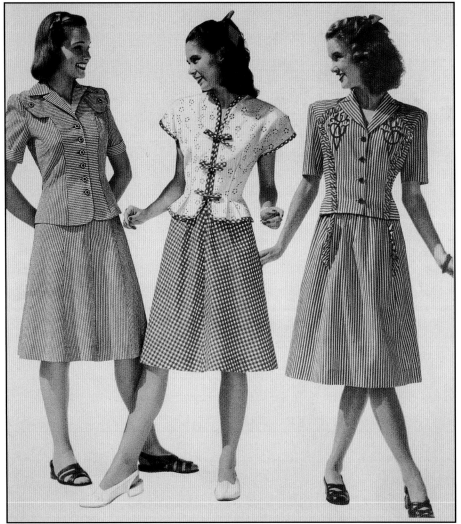

Bib front suit, woven-stripe seersucker two-piece, in tan and white, red and white, or blue and white. Bow-catcher, gingham, and eyelet two-piecer. Skirt has fullness at the waist. Jacket has peplum ripple, flirty gingham bow ties, and bias-checked banding all around, bright green and white or brown and white. Smart cotton two-piece charmer, jacket has vertical-striped panel front, horizontal striped sides and back. Ruffles and embroidery embellish outfit. Medium blue, medium brown, or red, all with white stripes. $5. [$20-30] *Spring/summer 1947*

For Sunday best or daily dress-up…two-color striped cotton seersucker, button-front, slimming and well tailored, in red and gray, red and navy, medium blue and navy, or brown and green stripes. Embroidered Sanforized cotton, frosty white stitched scroll embroidery, medium blue or medium green. One-piece looks like two-piece, becoming jacket front effect on attractive print, with popcorn shirring and slim seven-gore skirt, medium blue or rose background print. $5. [$10-20] *Spring/summer 1947*

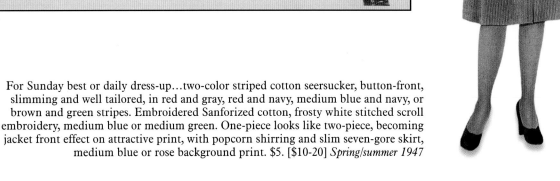

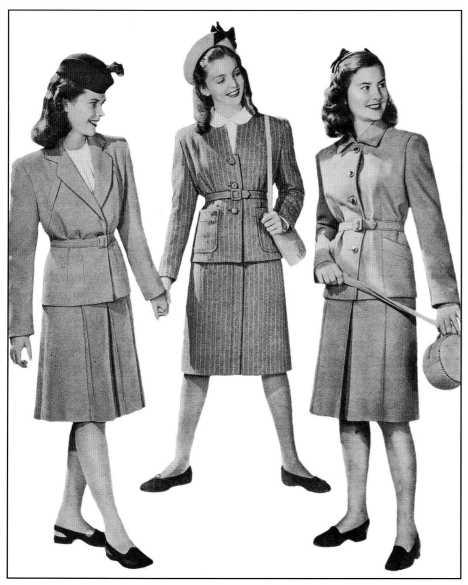

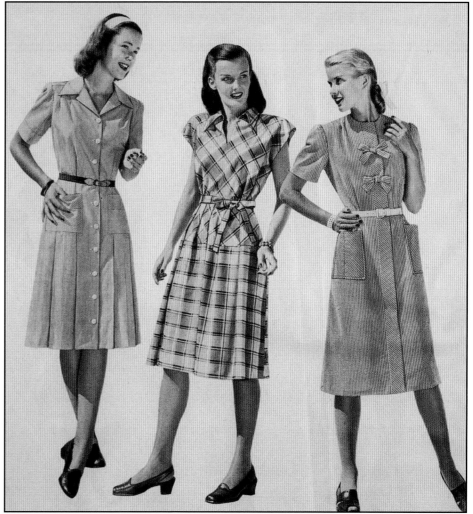

Sears Honeylanes…blaze a fashion trail for teens in suits this year! Shetland-type all wool dressmaker suit, mint or cocoa. Chalk stripe suit in menswear, gray all wool suiting, wear with or without self belt. New shirtwaist suit in all wool flannel. Flange shoulders, wide sleeves, and button-up collar, in light blue, medium gold, or coral. $13-16. [$15-20] *Spring/summer 1947*

Quality cotton dresses show off a young figure. Preshrunk Lonsdale chambray, woven stripes on white, non-gap button-front, in red, brown, lavender, medium green, or medium blue stripes. Woven block plaid gingham, young and sleeveless with pointed layback collar, pink or light blue ground plaid. Seersucker stripes on white ground, round collarless neckline, bias stripes, and two accent bows, in red and gray, red and navy, medium blue and navy, or brown and green. $5. [$10-20] *Spring/summer 1947*

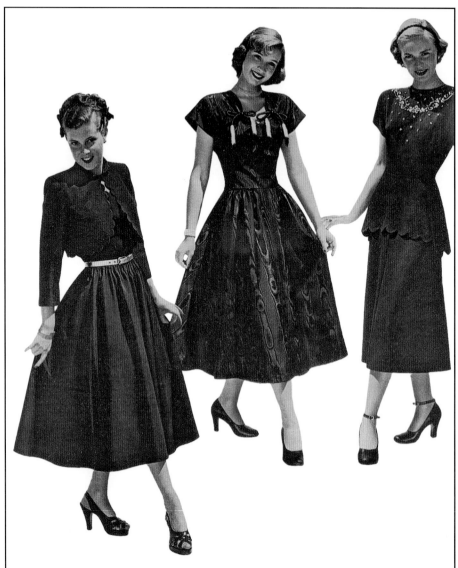

Dress and bolero…rayon faille, for very special dates…an adorable dress with a big 110-inch skirt and a little nipped waist, gold color belt. For afternoon and street wear, a wonderful bolero ensemble, in black, turquoise, or dark green. Real ermine tails, big 115-inch skirt, crisp, handsomely self-patterned rayon moiré with fine detail, in black or dark brown. Twinkling turquoise and gold sequins on mossy-textured rayon crepe, scalloped peplum dips and flares to give an exciting silhouette. Black or dark brown. $13-14. [$10-20] *Fall/winter 1948*

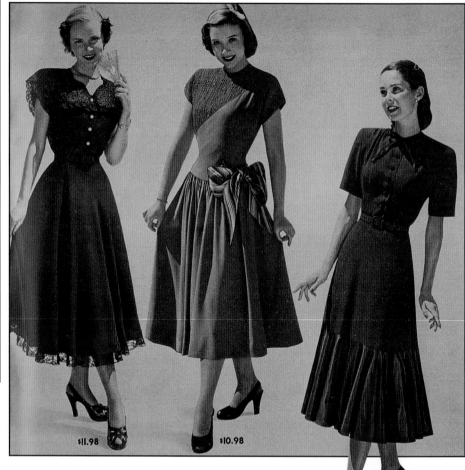

$11.98 $10.98

Pretty matching lace on fine rayon alpaca, buttons of sparkling rhinestones set in gold, fine cotton lace, in turquoise, winter rose, or black. Smoothly molded bodice and big roman-striped rayon taffeta bow accent 100-inch skirt, gathered all around, in black or deep blue. Wonderful flared flounce, rayon alpaca with circular-cut, neck binding, with bow tie and buttons of matching rayon taffeta, in dark brown or black. $11-12. [$10-20] *Fall/winter 1948*

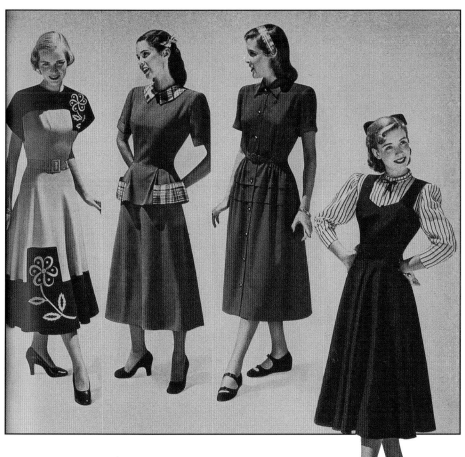

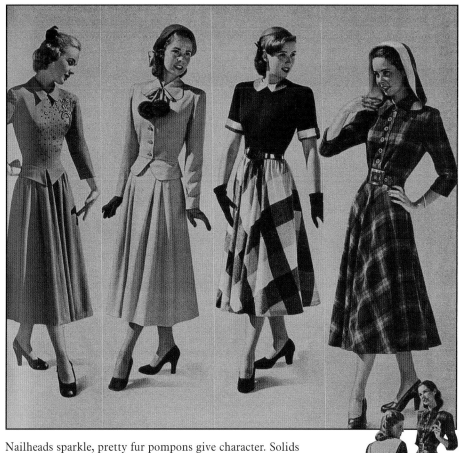

Faille-ribbed rayon…crisp, pretty, and looks expensive! Flaring flounce with applied design, looks like embroidery, in beige with dark brown or aqua blue with black. Two-piece smooth fitting top with flaring peplum, pockets and cuffs are crisp rayon taffeta in a bright woven plaid, in black, navy blue, or Kelly green. Button-front, easy to slip into, comfortable and easy to wash, in violet, aqua blue, and lipstick red. Low-cut jumper with 110-inch skirt, with blouse to contrast. Black jumper with pink and black, or light blue and black spun rayon blouse. $8-9. [$15-20] *Fall/winter 1948*

Nailheads sparkle, pretty fur pompons give character. Solids and plaids, in warm wool and rayon blends. One and two-piece dresses give style and comfort. $8-14. [$10-20] *Fall/winter 1948*

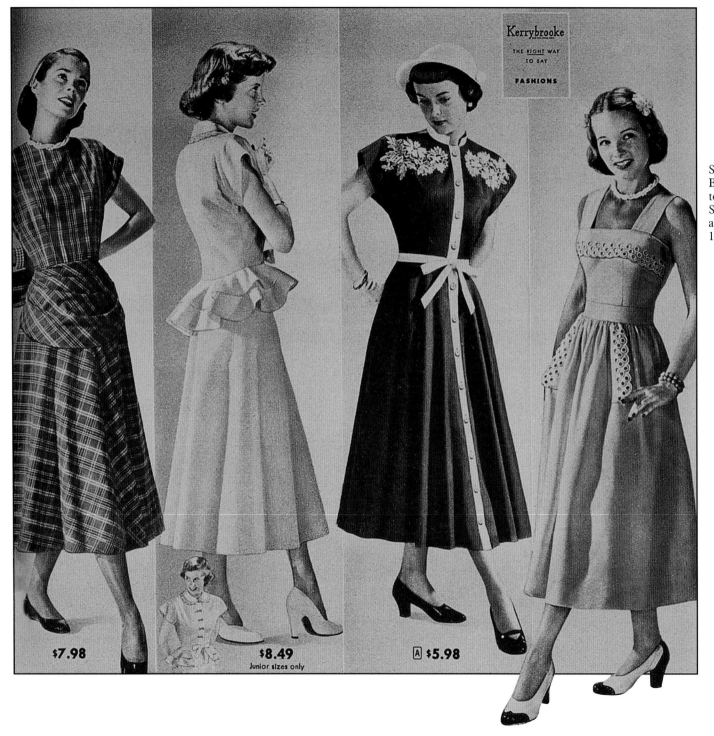

Kerrybrooke

THE RIGHT WAY
TO SAY

FASHIONS

$7.98

$8.49
Junior sizes only

Ⓐ $5.98

Sanforized gingham…very fine and soft. Beautiful styles, lovely to look at, wonderful to wear. Preshrunk waffle pique and Sanforized broadcloth styles. Colorful plaids and soft, fresh solids for summer. $7-9. [$10-15] *Spring/summer 1949*

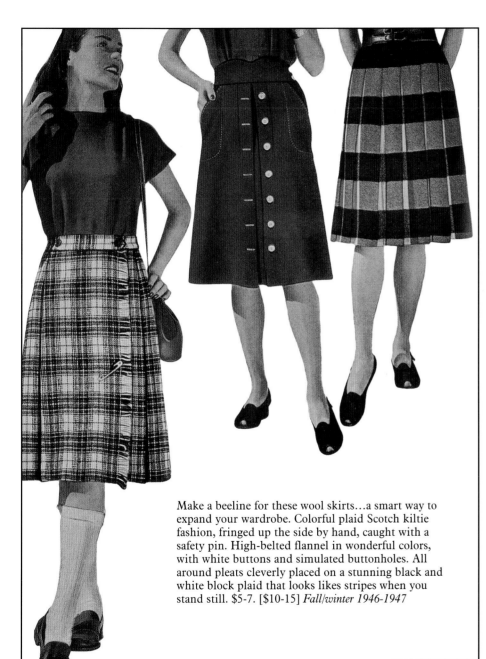

Make a beeline for these wool skirts…a smart way to expand your wardrobe. Colorful plaid Scotch kiltie fashion, fringed up the side by hand, caught with a safety pin. High-belted flannel in wonderful colors, with white buttons and simulated buttonholes. All around pleats cleverly placed on a stunning black and white block plaid that looks likes stripes when you stand still. $5-7. [$10-15] *Fall/winter 1946-1947*

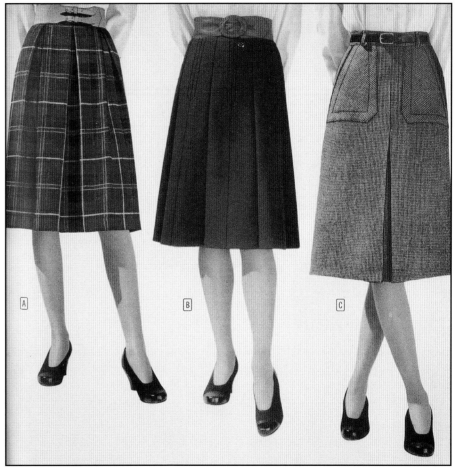

One smart skirt makes many changes…choose wool or part wool to team with sweaters or blouses. Plaids, solids, and checks, with attractive lines, young and new. $4-6. [$10-15] *Fall/winter 1946-1947*

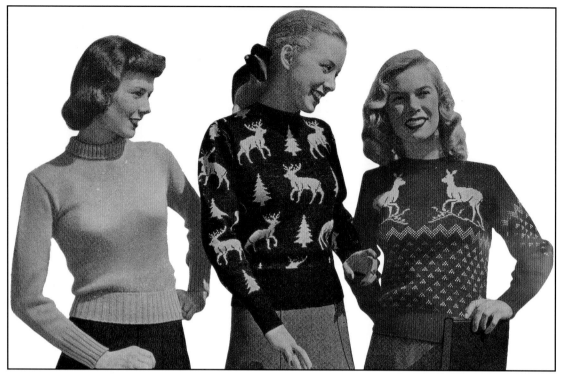

Top ski pants, skating togs, or casual skirts with gay Kerrybrooke pullovers. Fitted sweaters with low turtle neckline, in gray, black, or white. Jacquard sportster with casual lines and color combinations as Norwegian classics. Navy blue or red with white. $4-7. [$20-30] *Fall/winter 1946-1947*

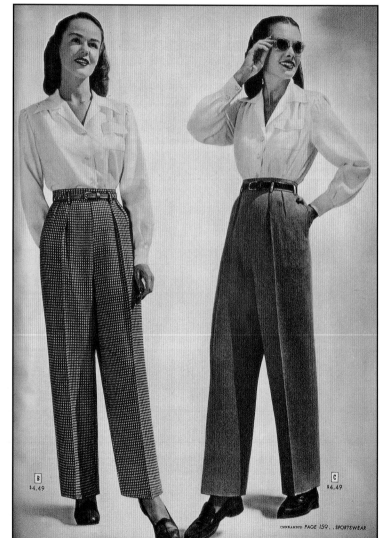

Kerrybrookes are the American woman's ideal slacks, man-tailored, beautifully fitting, and cut for action. Checked part wool, in black and white or brown and white. Menswear gray in a splendid blend. $4-5. [$10-20] *Fall/winter 1946-1947*

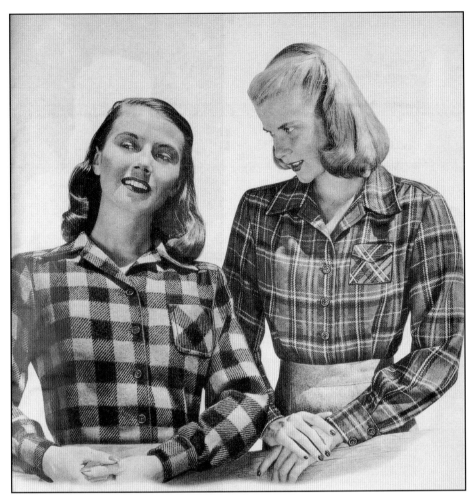

No need to borrow your brother's…here's your own loud plaid shirt! Block plaid all wool or Scotch plaid part wool, wear for warmth, fun for school or sports. Black and red, black and white, or red, blue and white plaid combinations. $4-6. [$10-20] *Fall/winter 1946-1947*

Coat sweaters in V-neck or collar styles are the choice of value-minded women for warmth, comfort, and serviceability. All wool V-necks and Shaker sweaters, in navy, maroon, or wine. $2-6. [$15-20] *Fall/winter 1946-1947*

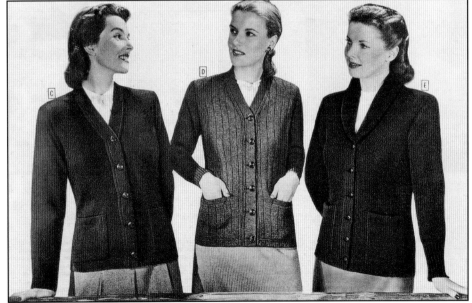

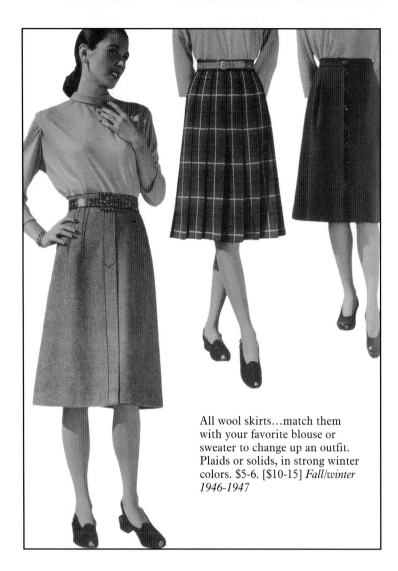

All wool skirts…match them with your favorite blouse or sweater to change up an outfit. Plaids or solids, in strong winter colors. $5-6. [$10-15] *Fall/winter 1946-1947*

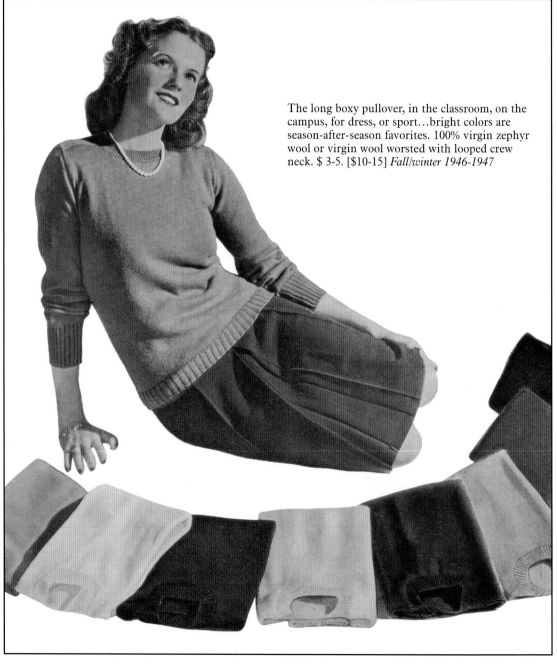

The long boxy pullover, in the classroom, on the campus, for dress, or sport…bright colors are season-after-season favorites. 100% virgin zephyr wool or virgin wool worsted with looped crew neck. $ 3-5. [$10-15] *Fall/winter 1946-1947*

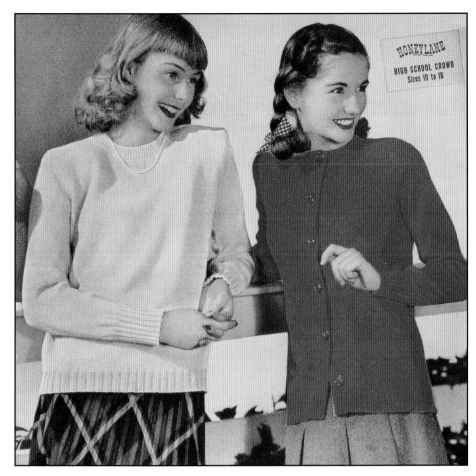

Honeylane all wool classics, casual boxy pullover or classic boxy cardigan in three qualities, in bright red, yellow, medium blue, or dark green. $2-4. [$20-30] *Fall/winter 1946-1947*

Youthful all wool "Go Togethers" in newest fitted styles, versatile, casually worn or tucked into a skirt with a big belt. Hip-length, short sleeve, and long sleeve pullovers. In aqua, red, yellow, gray, pink, black, brown, or dark green. $2-4. [$10-15] *Fall/winter 1946-1947*

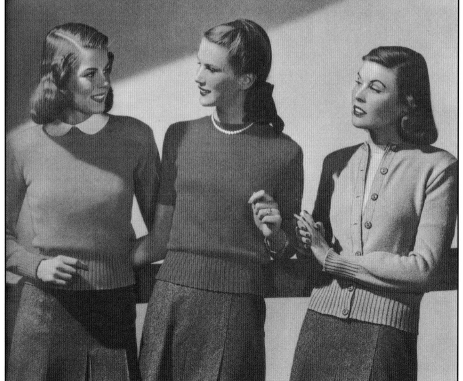

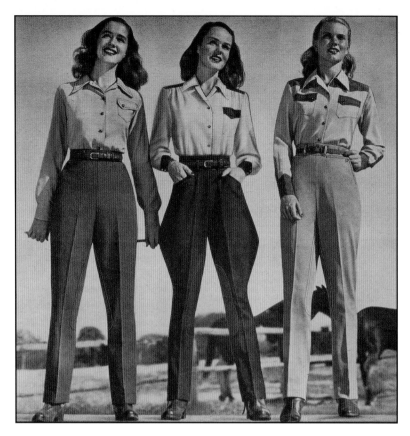

Figure flattering riding togs…Western styled for dude ranch or prairie wear. Denim frontier style pants, rayon gabardine shirt, Sanforized mercerized cotton gabardine jodhpurs, two-tone rayon riding shirt, and gabardine frontier pants. $3-7. [$10-15] *Fall/winter 1946-1947*

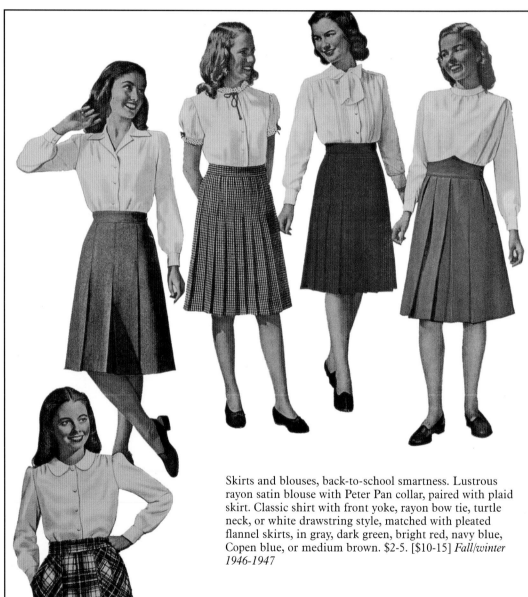

Skirts and blouses, back-to-school smartness. Lustrous rayon satin blouse with Peter Pan collar, paired with plaid skirt. Classic shirt with front yoke, rayon bow tie, turtle neck, or white drawstring style, matched with pleated flannel skirts, in gray, dark green, bright red, navy blue, Copen blue, or medium brown. $2-5. [$10-15] *Fall/winter 1946-1947*

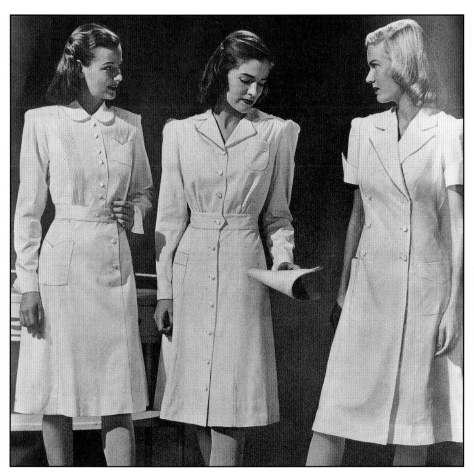

Right for your job…fresh, smartly tailored cottons and rayons for lab, beauty parlor, or doctor's office. Peter Pan collar and cluster tucking from shoulder to waist, popular button-front, or double breasted coat styles. White or medium bluc. $3-5. [$10-15] *Fall/winter 1946-1947*

Sears Honeylanes, most popular slacks in America for teens. Man-tailored for the young figure. Menswear gray in wool blends, part wool buffalo check shirt, in red and black or white and black. Finest flannel slacks, virgin wool, in dark brown or navy blue. 100% virgin wool sweater, in yellow, white, gray, yellow, medium blue, bright red, or dark brown. $4-5. [$10-15] *Fall/winter 1946-1947*

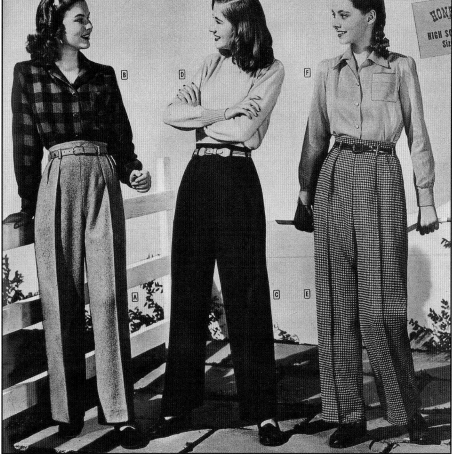

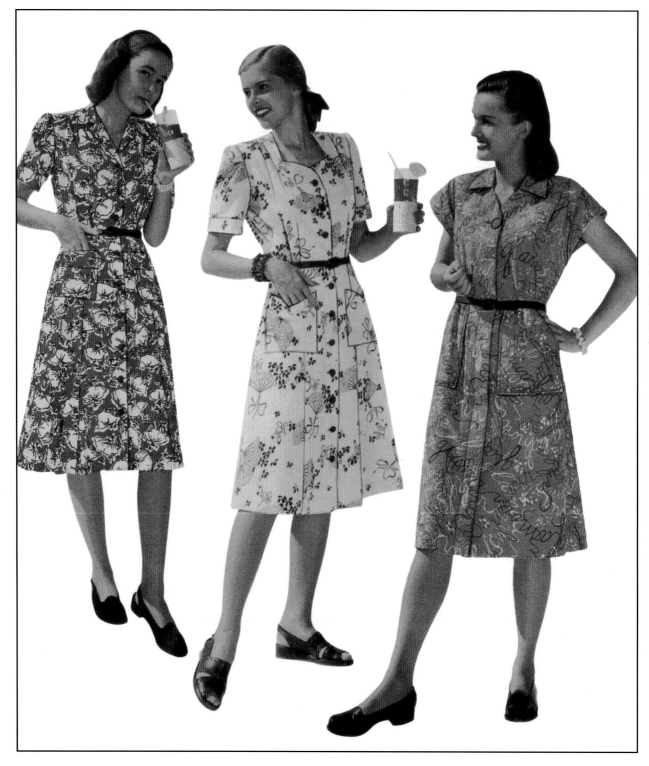

Printed cotton seersucker
button-front classics by
Colette. Ballerina print with
casual shirt style collar, pen-
and-ink print with curved
patch pockets and sweetheart
neck, or glamour print with
fly front that conceals its
buttons. $5. [$10-15] *Spring/
summer 1947*

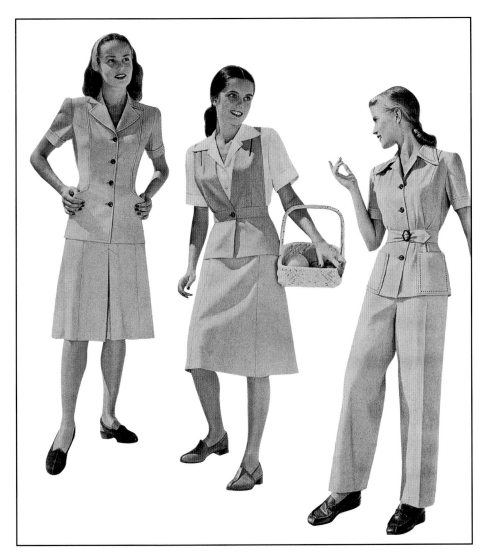

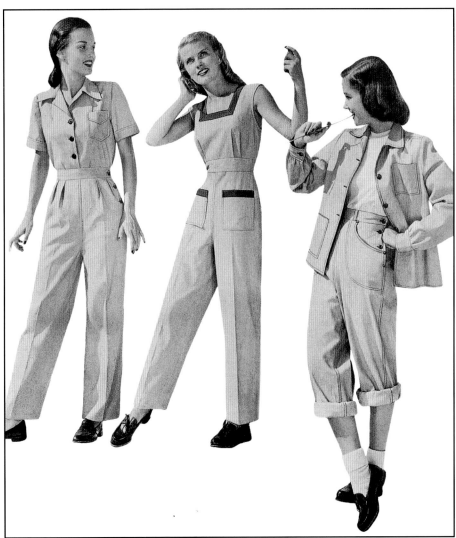

So smart, so right for town or sports. Kerrybrooke denim outfits, two-piece skirt or slack suit. Trim, young, and smart, well-tailored and figure-enhancing. Light blue or navy. $2-6. [$15-20] *Spring/summer 1947*

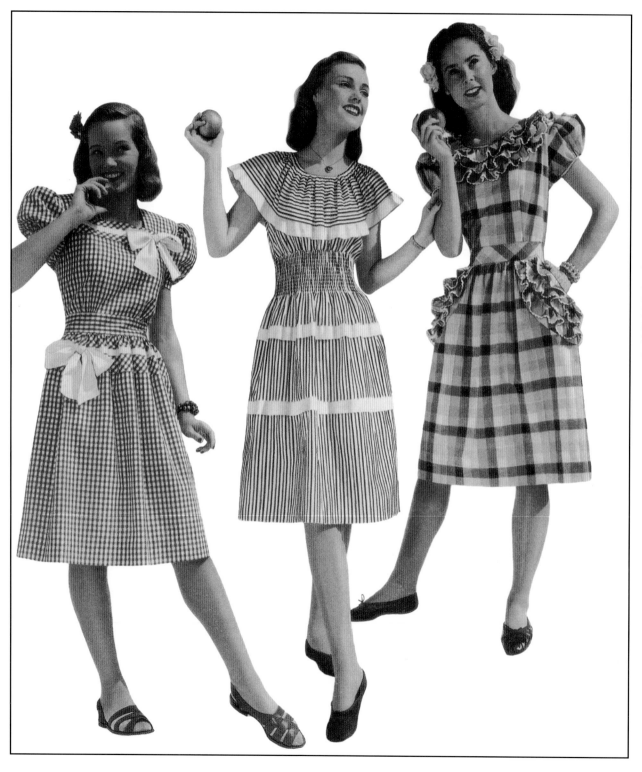

Wonderful cotton dresses with swingy skirts and slim tops. Checked gingham with king-sized bows, printed seersucker with Big Bertha collar, or plaid gingham with ruffles at shoulder and pockets, all Kerrybrooke fresh and fun. $5. [$10-15] *Spring/summer 1947*

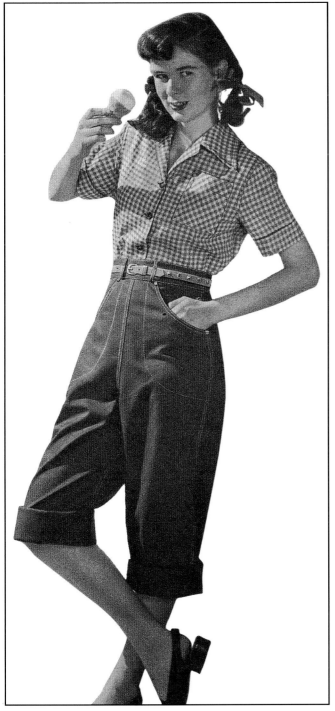

Denim dungarees, top fashion for sports and play, sturdy and long-wearing for work and roughing it, in navy blue. $3. [$10-20] Checked cotton mannish shirt, red and white check. $2. [$5-10] *Spring/summer 1947*

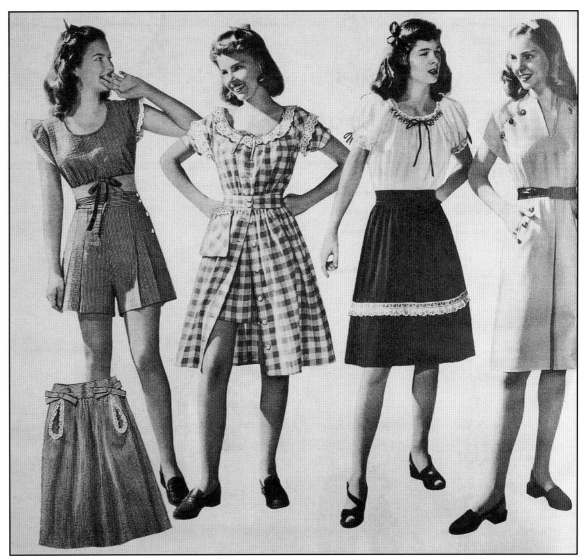

Enchanting playclothes for every fun-loving hour. Two-piece midriff playsuit of striped cotton seersucker, checked cotton playsuit and skirt, black dirndl peasant skirt in Sanforized cotton, with white peasant-style drawstring blouse with balloon sleeves in rayon. $3-6. [$10-15] *Spring/summer 1947*

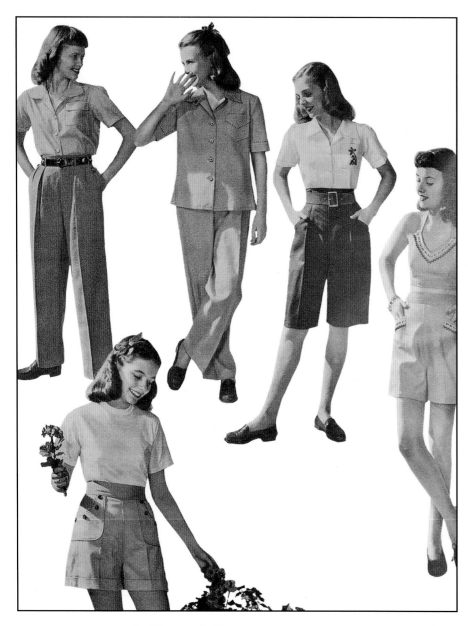

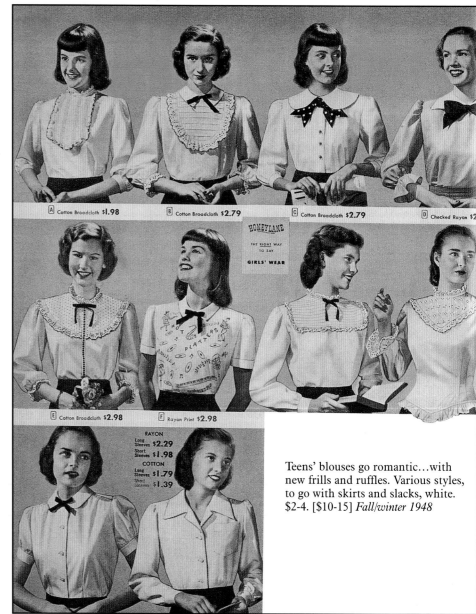

Teen sports togs with glamour looks and sturdy wear. Classic boy shorts, slacks, denim slack suit, pedal pushers, and two-piece cotton twill bra set, in lively summer colors, including yellow, Copen blue, or bright red. $2-6. [$5-10] *Spring/summer 1947*

A Cotton Broadcloth $1.98   B Cotton Broadcloth $2.79   C Cotton Broadcloth $2.79   D Checked Rayon $2

HONEYLANE
THE RIGHT WAY TO SAY
GIRLS' WEAR

E Cotton Broadcloth $2.98   F Rayon Print $2.98

RAYON
Long Sleeves $2.29
Short Sleeves $1.98
COTTON
Long Sleeves $1.79
Short Sleeves $1.39

Teens' blouses go romantic…with new frills and ruffles. Various styles, to go with skirts and slacks, white. $2-4. [$10-15] *Fall/winter 1948*

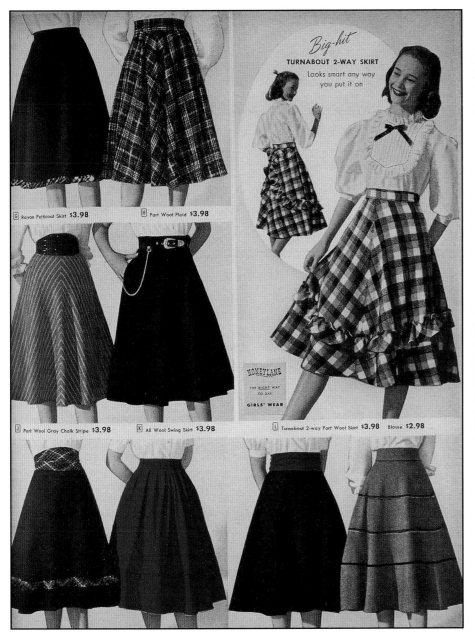

Big-hit
TURNABOUT 2-WAY SKIRT
Looks smart any way you put it on

HONEYLANE
THE RIGHT WAY TO SAY
GIRLS' WEAR

G Rayon Petticoat Skirt $3.98   H Part Wool Plaid $3.98

J Part Wool Gray Chalk Stripe $3.98   K All Wool Swing Skirt $3.98   L Turnabout 2-way Part Wool Skirt $3.98   Blouse $2.98

Honeylane skirts. Styles include rayon petticoat, part wool plaid, turnabout two-way, part wool gray chalk stripe, all wool swing skirt, all wool plaid 'n'plain, rayon flounce, wool cummerbund, or gray wool swing skirts. $4-5. [$10-15] *Fall/ winter 1948*

Denim playclothes, overalls in yellow or navy blue, denim sunsuit in multicolor stripes, denim and checked outfit, pedal pushers trimmed with red and white checked cotton, pedal pushers, in red, navy, or light blue. $2-3. [$5-10] *Spring/summer 1949*

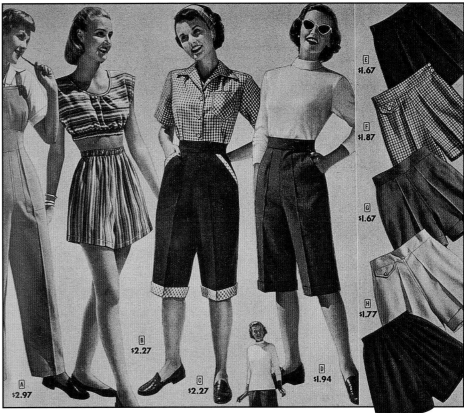

E $1.67
F $1.87
G $1.67
H $1.77

A $2.97
B $2.27
C $2.27
D $1.94

93

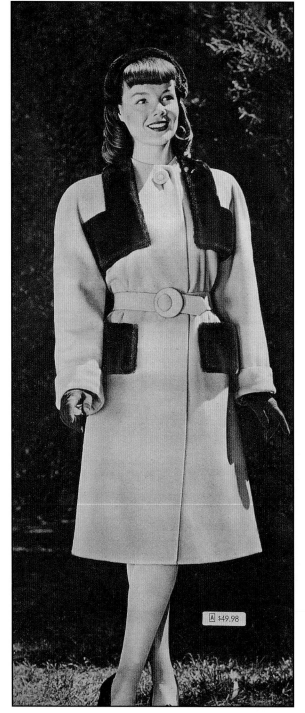

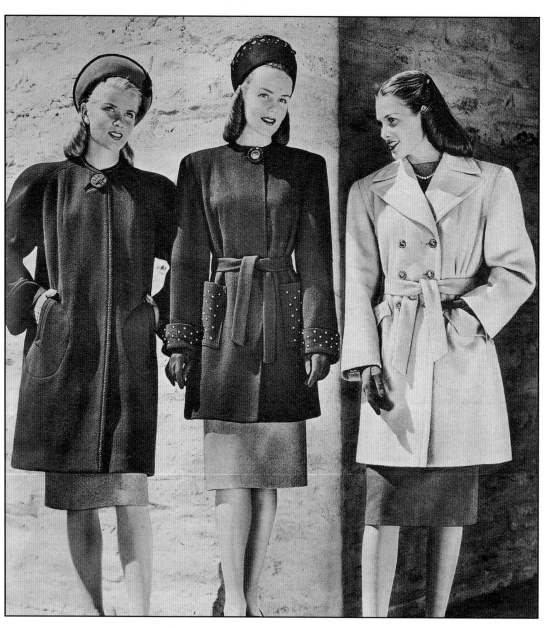

A $49.98

The dressy shortcoat in soft-draping all wool, in black, dark brown, winter white, or wine. Glitter coat is showered with nailheads, its fullness smartly caught in with a belt, in black, royal, winter white, or wine. The double-breasted coat in fluffy woven wool fleece, in black, dark brown, winter white, or Kelly green. $20-25. [$20-30] *Fall/winter 1946-1947*

Beaver-dyed mouton lamb on a coat of suede-soft all wool, squares of bolero fashion on top, covers pockets below smartly-belted waist. Dark brown, medium green, medium blue, or royal blue. $50. [$20-30] *Fall/winter 1946-1947*

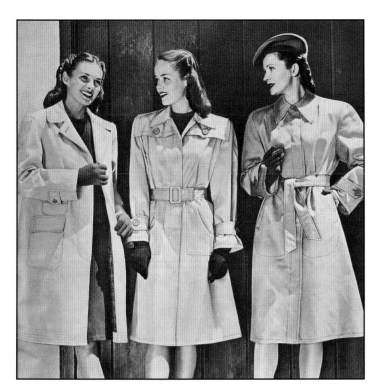

Sun or shower coats, smartly styled fly-front raincoat, nice and boxy, in medium tan. The Hollywood coat, with attractive swaggery collar and roomy armholes, in medium tan. Women's special, a fashion-wise coat smartly adapted for larger sizes, in medium tan or navy blue. $5-12. [$15-20] *Fall/winter 1946-1947*

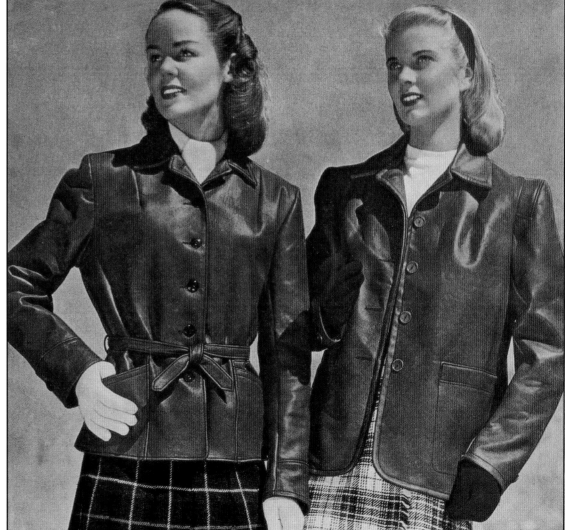

Warm capeskin for school belles or sports fans, belted or boxy with hold-everything pockets. Medium brown or black capeskin. $14-16. [$30-40] *Fall/winter 1946-1947*

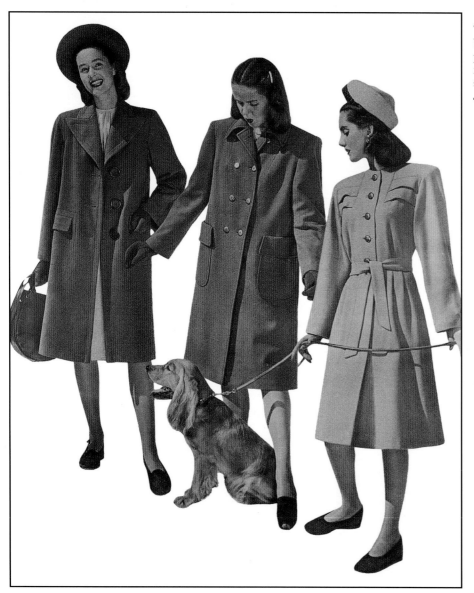

The important boy coat, wonderful all wool, wide welt seaming, in medium blue, gray, coral, or black. Double-file buttons, shiny as new pennies, on a perky shirt, collared. Casual all wool, in medium blue, gray, Kelly green, or medium brown. The fit-and-flare coat has your pet cardigan neckline and shutter tucks, in medium blue, gray, Kelly green, or black. $20. [$20-30] *Spring/summer 1947*

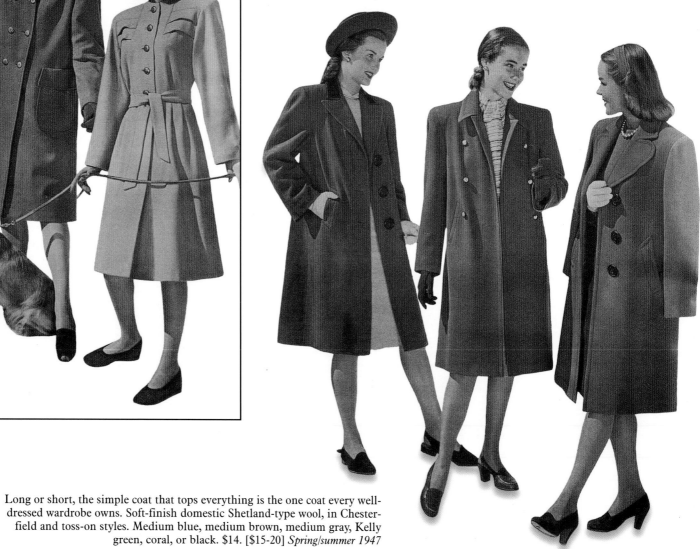

Long or short, the simple coat that tops everything is the one coat every well-dressed wardrobe owns. Soft-finish domestic Shetland-type wool, in Chesterfield and toss-on styles. Medium blue, medium brown, medium gray, Kelly green, coral, or black. $14. [$15-20] *Spring/summer 1947*

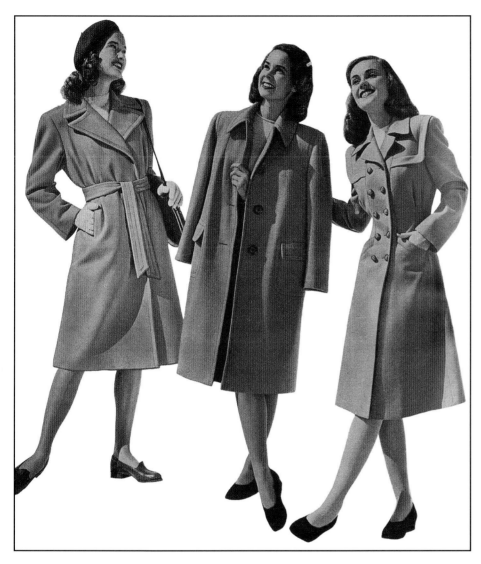

The dashing polo coat, deep-downy suede-soft all wool, in light gray, medium blue, or Kelly green. Shirt-collar coat, truly classic in every detail, in beige tan, medium brown, or Kelly green. Button-tight look, yoke squares off smartly, collar is carefully notched, in navy blue, medium blue, or Kelly green. $20. [$20-30] *Spring/summer 1947*

Stunning stripes in white and red take turns on popular menswear gray all wool flannel match-ups. Contrasts, the newest fashion flash, dominate this rayon-lined shortcoat, in black and white or brown and white. $17. [$10-20] *Spring/summer 1947*

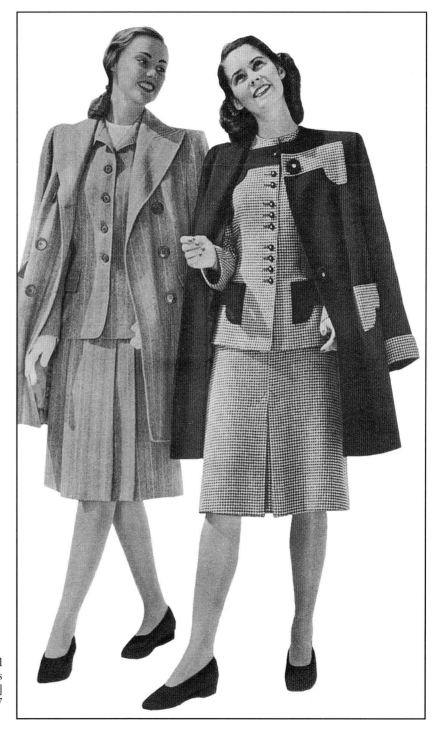

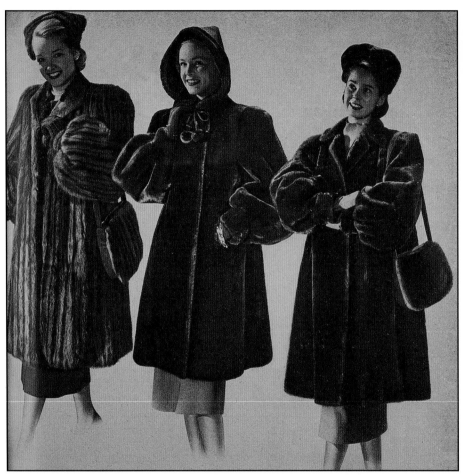

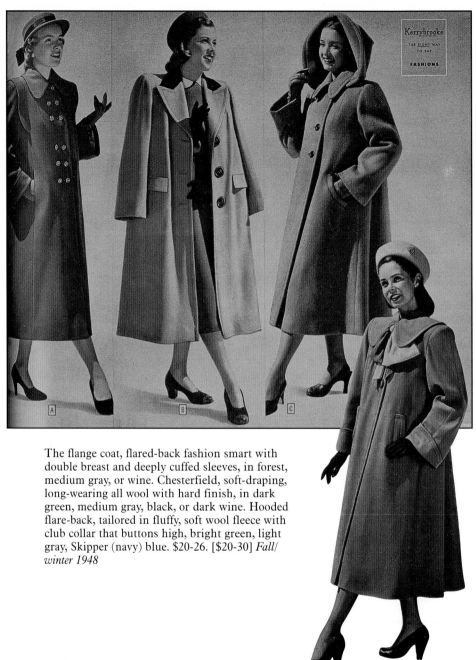

Stunning, three-piece ensemble: Luxurious coat, halo hat, and zipper bag. Coney-dyed the tawny brown of wild mink. $70. Detachable hood, young 3/4-length Kerrybrooke coat of Beaver-dyed mouton lamb, plastic-processed to resist water. $95. Lush, beaver brown dyed mouton lamb three-piece outfit. $95. [$60-85] *Fall/winter 1948*

The flange coat, flared-back fashion smart with double breast and deeply cuffed sleeves, in forest, medium gray, or wine. Chesterfield, soft-draping, long-wearing all wool with hard finish, in dark green, medium gray, black, or dark wine. Hooded flare-back, tailored in fluffy, soft wool fleece with club collar that buttons high, bright green, light gray, Skipper (navy) blue. $20-26. [$20-30] *Fall/winter 1948*

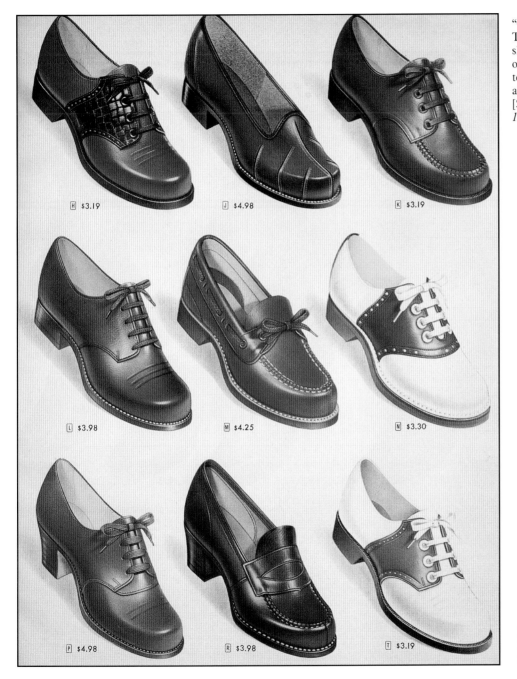

H $3.19 J $4.98 K $3.19

L $3.98 M $4.25 N $3.30

P $4.98 R $3.98 T $3.19

"Out of this World" Teenright styles, hep cats, shankmasters, moc style, oxford sharpies, and the teen favorite, saddle style, all in brown leather. $3-4. [$5-10] *Fall/winter 1946-1947*

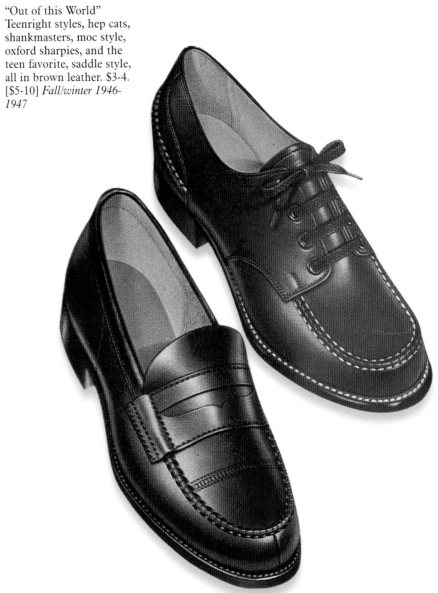

Larky footnotes to schoolday casuals…sparky slip-ons, leather sole and heel, in brown. Madcap twosomes, oxfords with moc-type vamp, leather insole, sole, and rubber heel, brown leather. $3-5. [$5-10] *Fall/winter 1946-1947*

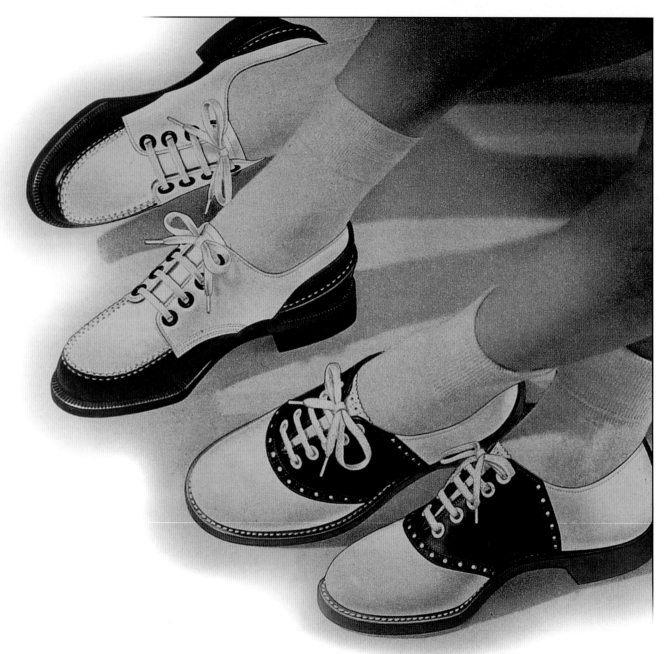

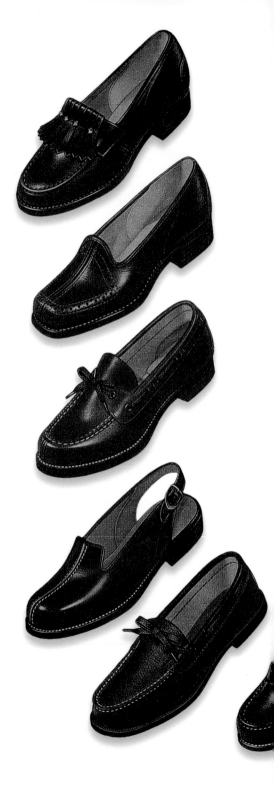

For buzzin' around to class or date, "Little Boy" saddles, moc-type smarties with
Kerrybrooke 100% teenage styling. Brown and white in both styles, two qualities. $4-7.
[$5-10] *Spring/summer 1947*

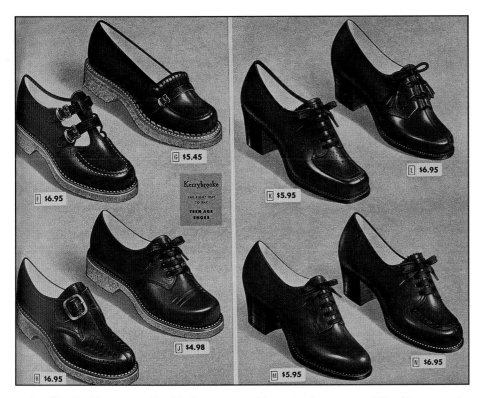

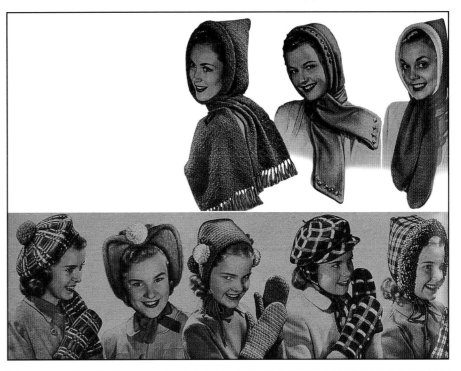

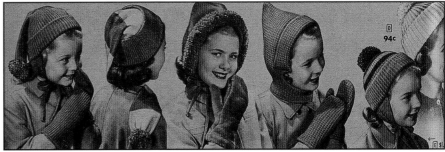

Put "Spring" in your walk with these crepe rubber soles for teenagers! Double strapped sandal, casual slip-on style, sport-time smarties. $5-7. [$5-10] *Fall/winter 1948*

Cozy and colorful warm-ups, stocking caps, bonnets, and mittens, for the cold, blustery winters. In warm, rich colors. $1-3. [$3-5] *Fall/winter 1948*

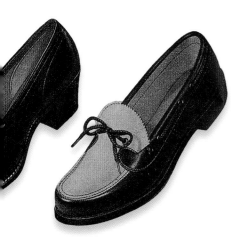

Larky young carefrees with a teenage point of view…smooth , simple and casual. Slip on moc-types, blithe shanksmares, and sling-back flatties. Dress 'em up or wear 'em casual. Brown leather. $3-6. [$5-10] *Spring/summer 1947*

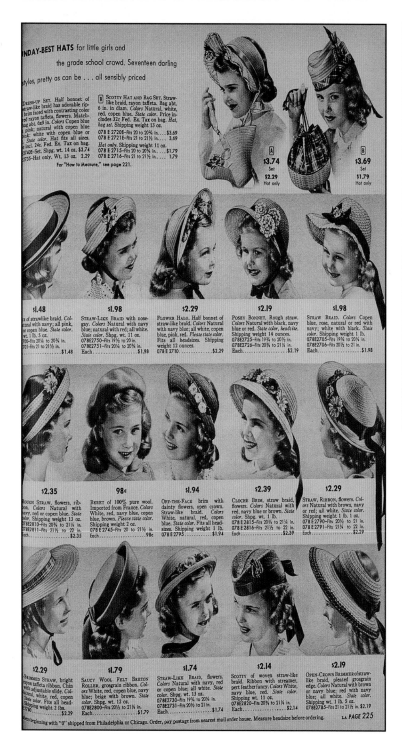

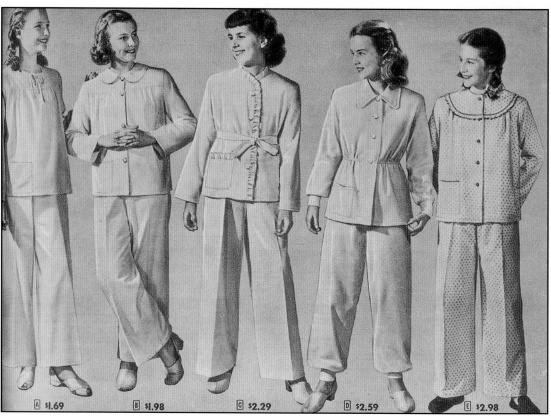

A $1.69 B $1.98 C $2.29 D $2.59 E $2.98

Warm flannelette pajamas for girls. Full-cut, slipover blouse in a boxy style with hanky pocket and trousers with an adjustable waistline. "Butcher boy" style with buttoned jacket. Feminine ruffle trim with belt. Ski-suit pajamas styled like sportswear with knit ski cuffs. Polka dot trimmed with ruffles and ric-rac for that charming, "old-fashioned" look. Honeylane pajamas man-tailored or warm, vat-dyed Sanforized flannelette. $2-3. [$10-15] *Fall/winter 1948*

Sunday-best hats for little girls and the grade school crowd. Darling styles, pretty as can be. Straw-like braid bonnets and wide-brimmed hats, flowered halos and off-the-face brims. Lots of pretty colors. $1-4. [$5-10] *Spring/summer 1949*

Suits and Dress Wear

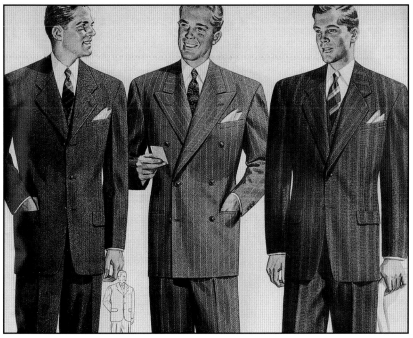

Exclusive Fashion Tailored 100% virgin wool worsted suits. Dignified stripe, single breasted. Chalk stripe, double breasted. Smart pattern, single breasted. In dark blue, dark gray, medium blue, medium brown, light blue, or light brown. $33. [$20-30] *Fall/winter 1946-1947*

These suits take the roughest, toughest, everyday wear, and come up looking neat, crisp, and "freshly tailored." Selected styles with vest. $27. [$20-30] *Fall/winter 1946-1947*

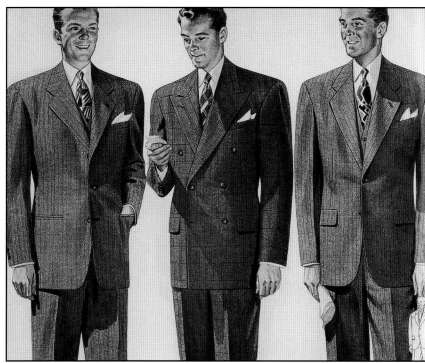

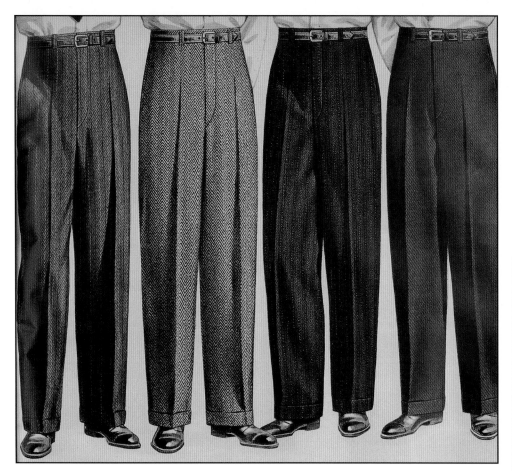

Conservative dress trousers. Hard finished, long-wearing fabrics, by Fashion Tailored. Part wool worsted, virgin wool herringbone, or 100% virgin wool worsted. Brown striped, blue striped, solid gray, or solid brown. $6-8. [$10-20] *Fall/winter 1946-1947*

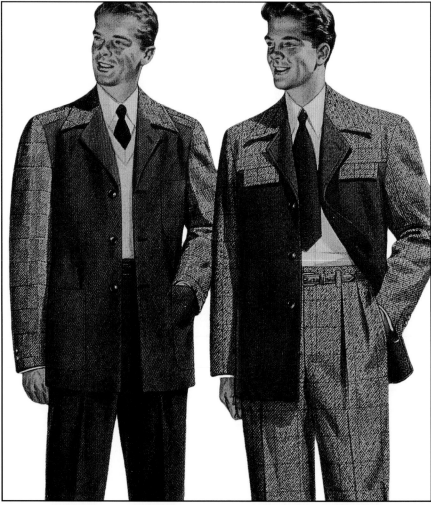

Wool-gabardine outfit, a leisure wear classic. Fancy check design on sleeves, collar, and back is dressy and easy in wearing comfort. Superbly styled outfit leads the sportswear parade. Smartly styled solid color coat has fancy novelty weave with a faint overplaid pattern on yoke, in blue or brown. $25-27. [$20-30] *Fall/winter 1946-1947*

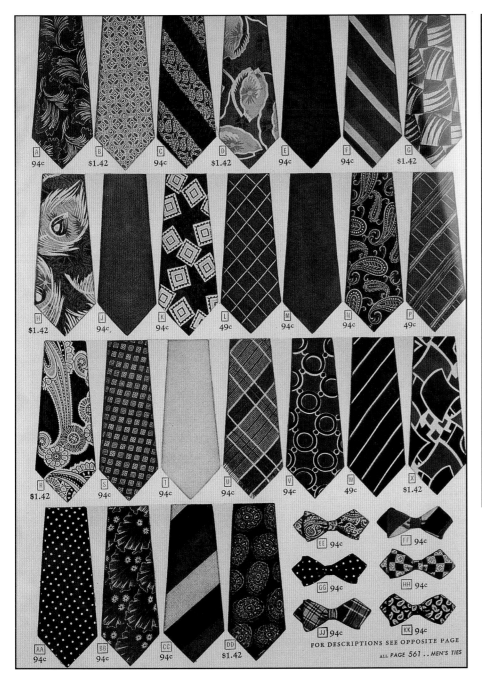

Pilgrim ties…rich colors, fun patterns, luxurious fabrics, wool interlined. $1-2. [$10-20]
Fall/winter 1946-1947

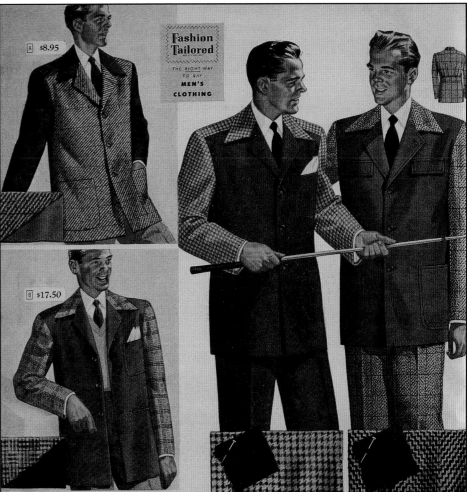

Wool and gabardine, enjoy the casual comfort. Virgin wool worsted coat that matches slacks, beautifully contrasted with a neat houndstooth check on collar, sleeves, and back. Brown or blue. Two-tone, dashingly styled coat with solid color, all wool front and lapels, overplaid pattern. $30. [$10-20] *Spring/summer 1947*

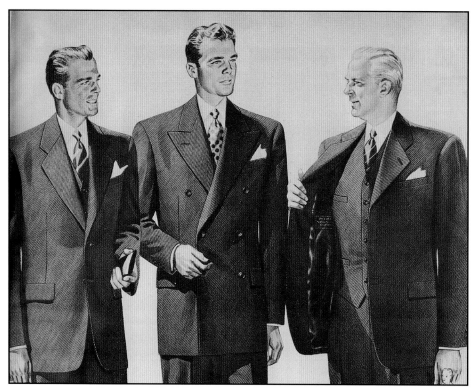

Fashion Tailored, heavyweight Serge, for men who like to dress well. Long-wearing twill weave fabric, hard finished, firmly textured, resists wrinkles. Navy blue or Oxford (dark) gray. $30-34. [$10-20] *Spring/summer 1947*

Popular gabardine with Fashion Tailored workmanship. Smart slacks with pleated and cuffed bottoms. In green, brown, tan, or blue. $7-8. [$5-10] *Spring/summer 1947*

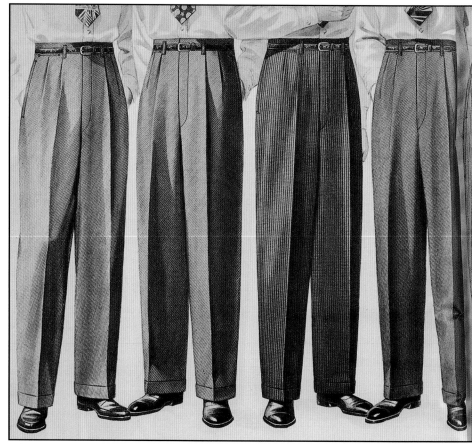

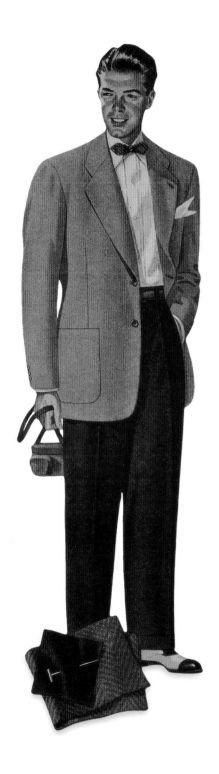

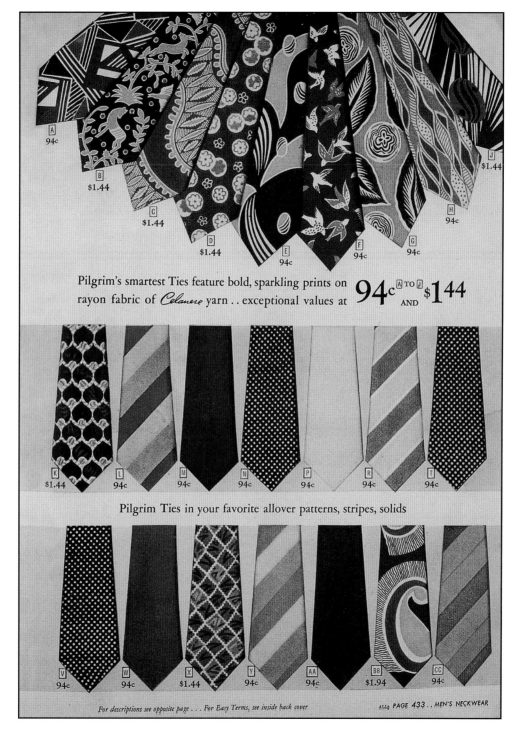

Pilgrim's smartest Ties feature bold, sparkling prints on rayon fabric of *Celanese* yarn .. exceptional values at **94c** A TO J **AND** **$1.44**

Pilgrim Ties in your favorite allover patterns, stripes, solids

For descriptions see opposite page . . . For Easy Terms, see inside back cover

ALLg PAGE 433 ., MEN'S NECKWEAR

LEFT · Sports coats and slacks...leisure time is pleasure time! Gay, sprightly shades, "featherweight," all wool glen plaid, herringbone, solid wool, and rayon sports coats, with gabardine or virgin wool flannel slacks. In camel tan, rust brown, dark brown, dark blue, or light blue, with complementing slacks. Two-piece outfit, $22-31. [$15-20] *Spring/summer 1947*

RIGHT · Pilgrim's smartest ties feature bold, sparkling prints on rayon fabric of Celanese yarn. Favorite allover patterns, stripes, and solids! $1-2. [$5-10] *Spring/summer 1947*

107

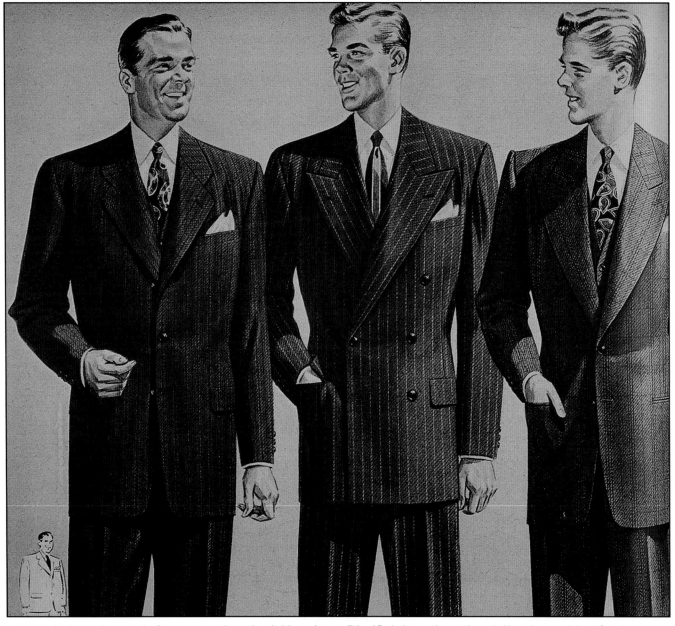

100% virgin wool worsteds. Strong, smooth, and wrinkle-resistant. Dignified alternating stripe, chalk stripe, or rich self-stripe with overplaid. Long-wearing, wrinkle-resistant, in medium gray, medium blue, or medium brown. $34. [$15-20] *Fall/winter 1948*

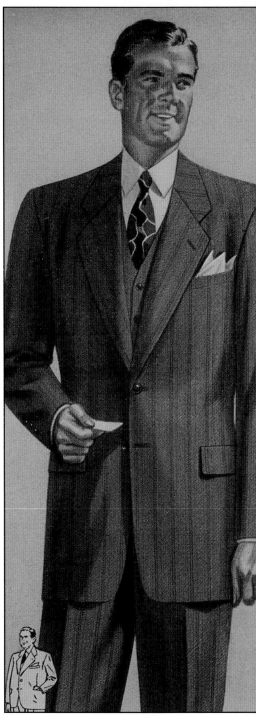

Expertly tailored 100% wool worsted suits for long service, perfect fit. $39. [$20-30] *Fall/winter 1948*

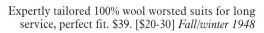

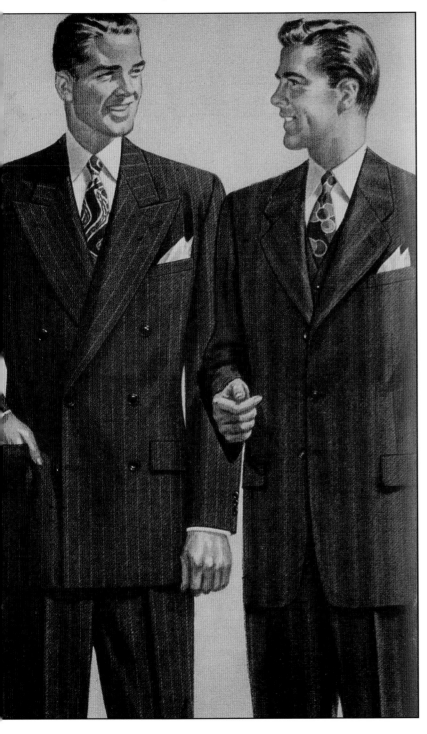

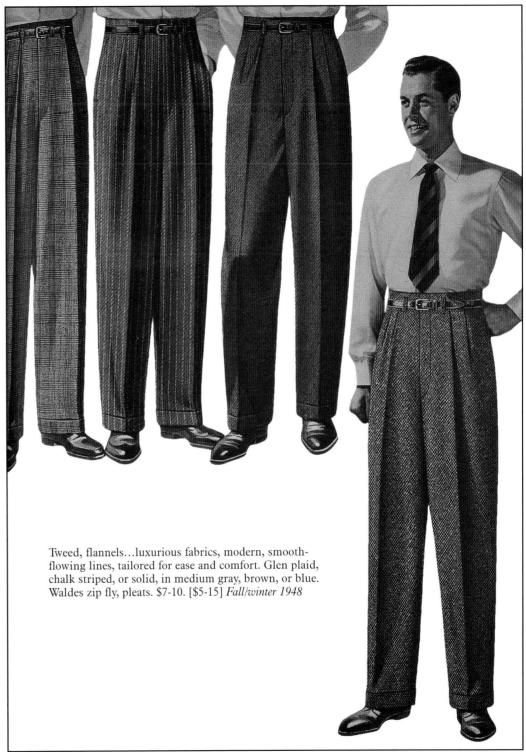

Tweed, flannels…luxurious fabrics, modern, smooth-flowing lines, tailored for ease and comfort. Glen plaid, chalk striped, or solid, in medium gray, brown, or blue. Waldes zip fly, pleats. $7-10. [$5-15] *Fall/winter 1948*

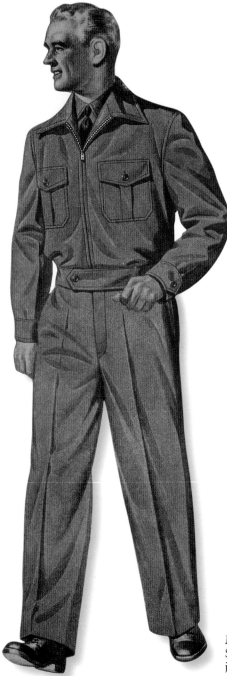

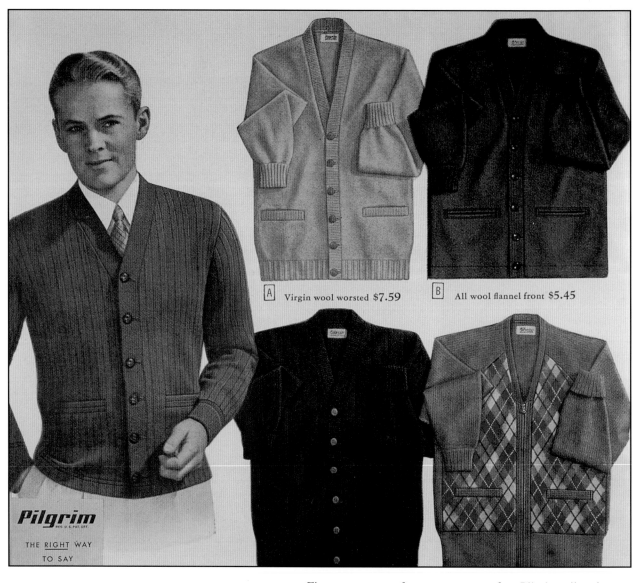

A — Virgin wool worsted $7.59

B — All wool flannel front $5.45

Mountain cloth post-war work outfit. Army-developed Sanforized material, in suntan, cocoa tan, or gray blue, jacket. Shirt with dress style collar, and pants for the hard-working man. $5-7. [$5-10] *Fall/winter 1946-1947*

Fine sweater coats for warm, easy comfort. Pilgrim tailored, fine zephyr wool, virgin wool worsted. Paneled rib effect style, argyle plaid with zipper front, and button-front, in camel tan, luggage brown, navy blue, or maroon. $4-8. [$15-10] *Fall/winter 1946-1947*

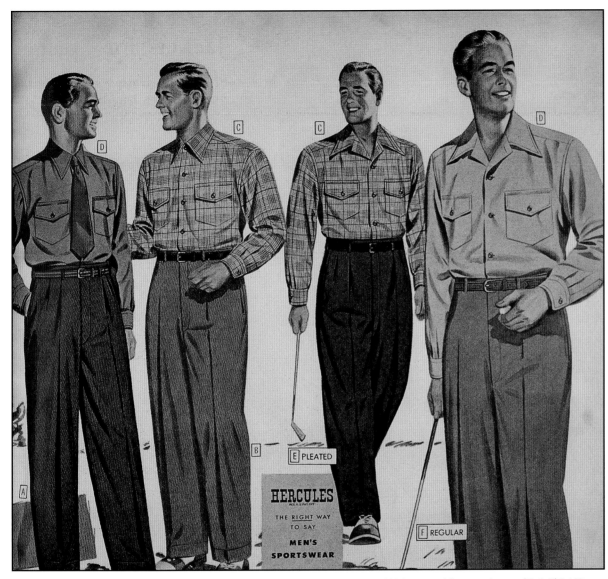

Hercules slacks and suits. Comfortable, carefree, and cool, in plaids or solid browns, blues, and tans. $3-4. [$5-10] *Spring/summer 1947*

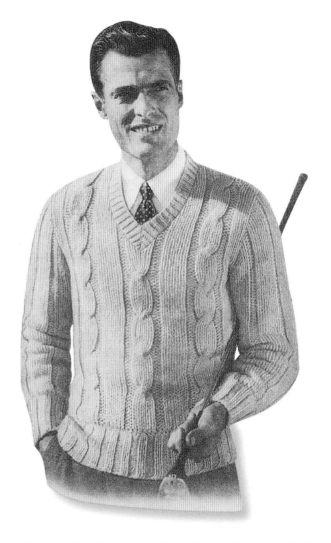

Sweaters for all casual wear, long sleeve pullover, panel rib effect, cable stitch, fine baby shaker stitch styles, warm and comfortable, grand with slacks. $3-6. [$15-20] *Spring/ summer 1947*

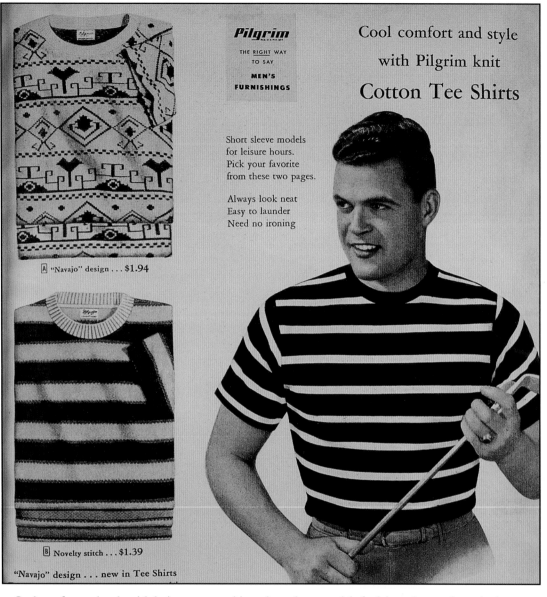

Pilgrim
THE RIGHT WAY
TO SAY
**MEN'S
FURNISHINGS**

Cool comfort and style
with Pilgrim knit
Cotton Tee Shirts

Short sleeve models
for leisure hours.
Pick your favorite
from these two pages.

Always look neat
Easy to launder
Need no ironing

[A] "Navajo" design . . . $1.94

[B] Novelty stitch . . . $1.39

"Navajo" design . . . new in Tee Shirts

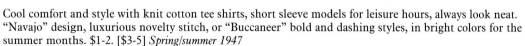

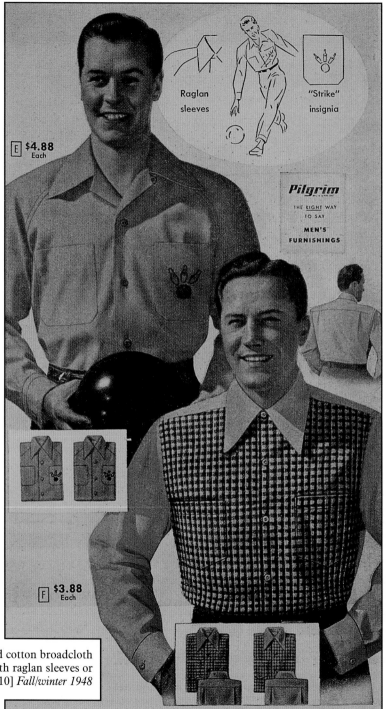

Raglan
sleeves

"Strike"
insignia

Pilgrim
THE RIGHT WAY
TO SAY
**MEN'S
FURNISHINGS**

[E] **$4.88**
Each

[F] **$3.88**
Each

Cool comfort and style with knit cotton tee shirts, short sleeve models for leisure hours, always look neat. "Navajo" design, luxurious novelty stitch, or "Buccaneer" bold and dashing styles, in bright colors for the summer months. $1-2. [$3-5] *Spring/summer 1947*

Long sleeve sports shirts, cotton poplin, pebbly rayon, and cotton broadcloth fabrics, in tans, blues, or greens. "Ten-pin" bowler style with raglan sleeves or plaid'n'plain style, all rayon fabric. $3-5. [$5-10] *Fall/winter 1948*

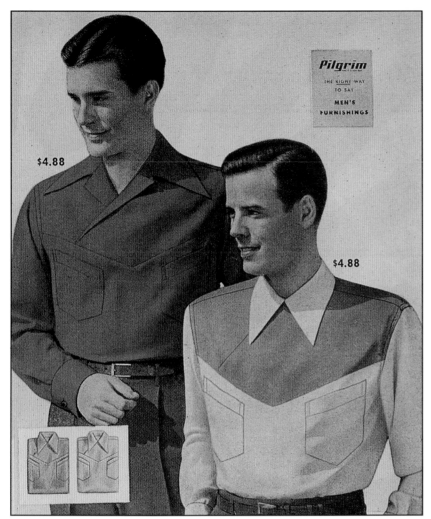

New deep yoke Pilgrim sports shirts, casual, cut-for-comfort style. Solid color vagabond, all rayon luana cloth, a close weave fabric with a fine cross rib. In blue, gray, or tan. Two-tone vagabond, double fabric yoke for longer wear with pleated back and sleeves, in bamboo (light tan) with medium tan yoke, or blue with a gray yoke. $5. [$10-15] *Fall/winter 1948*

New corduroy sportswear in rich, mellow shades. Reversible, campus, pile lined B-15 with mouton collar, or surcoat styles. $11-17. [$20-30] *Fall/winter 1948*

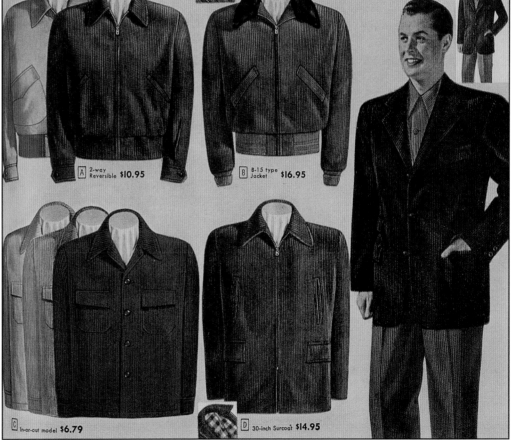

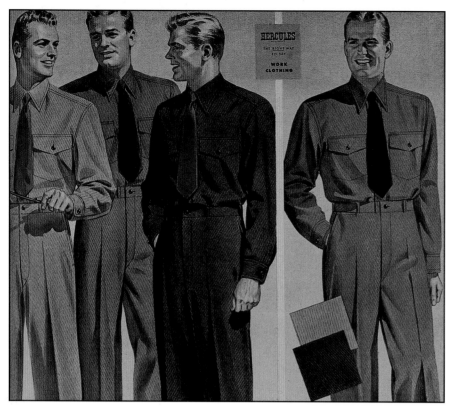

Sanforized twist twill pants, color matched twill shirts. Strong, boatsail drill pockets, vat-dyed, washfast and sunfast. Sturdy, comfortable, long-lasting. $3-5. [$10-15] *Fall/winter 1948*

Sweaters and tee shirts, casual coats and pullovers. Striped, cable stitched, plaid front, zipper or button, wool and cotton, in the best patterns and colors for fall. $4-6. [$15-20] *Fall/winter 1948*

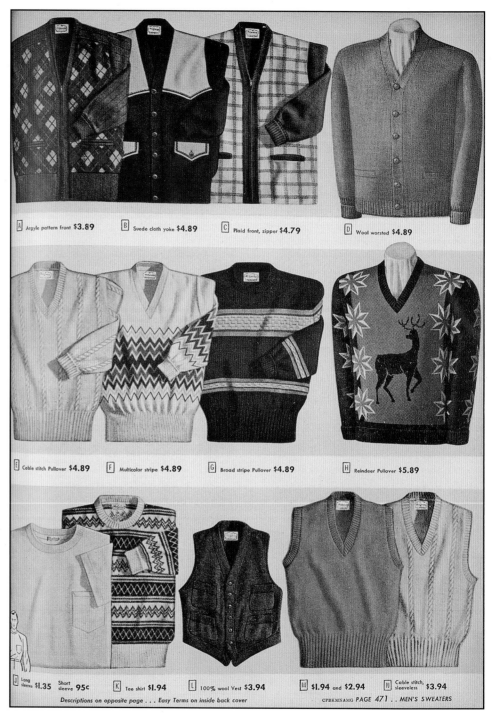

A Argyle pattern front $3.89   B Suede cloth yoke $4.89   C Plaid front, zipper $4.79   D Wool worsted $4.89

E Cable stitch Pullover $4.89   F Multicolor stripe $4.89   G Broad stripe Pullover $4.89   H Reindeer Pullover $5.89

J Long sleeve $1.35 Short sleeve 95c   K Tee shirt $1.94   L 100% wool Vest $3.94   M $1.94 and $2.94   N Cable stitch, sleeveless $3.94

Descriptions on opposite page . . . Easy Terms on inside back cover   CPBKMNAMG PAGE *471* . . MEN'S SWEATERS

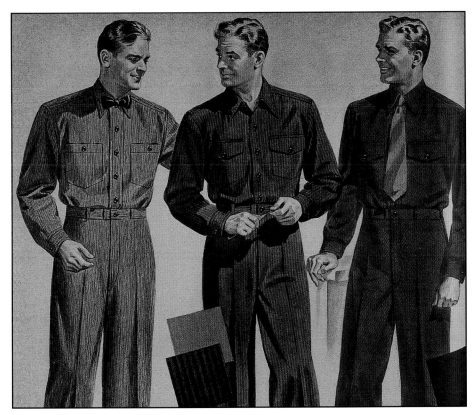

Hercules Sanforized outfits, oxford gray covert, drills and jeans, strong cotton yarns in herringbone pattern, and deep shade gabardine. Perfect fitting work clothing, extra looks of dress-type tailoring. $2-4. [$5-10] *Fall/winter 1948*

Pilgrim sports shirts, long sleeve styles. Three qualities: washfast cotton, smooth rayon, or all-rayon. Made for comfort. $3-5. [$10-15] *Fall/winter 1948*

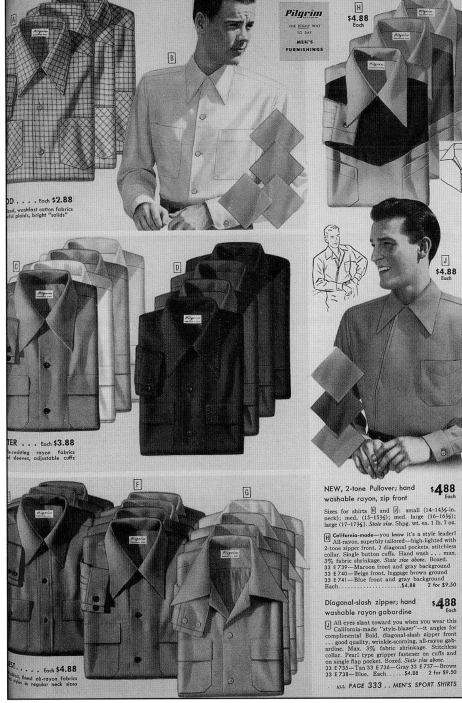

Pilgrim

THE RIGHT WAY
TO SAY

**MEN'S
FURNISHINGS**

[H] $4.88 Each

OD . . . . Each $2.88

zed, washfast cotton fabrics
rful plaids, bright "solids"

[J] $4.88 Each

TER . . . Each $3.88

e-resisting rayon fabrics
d sleeves, adjustable cuffs

EST . . . . Each $4.88

ed, finest all-rayon fabrics
styles in regular neck sizes

**NEW, 2-tone Pullover; hand
washable rayon, zip front** $4.88 Each

Sizes for shirts [H] and [J]: small (14-14½-in.
neck); med. (15-15½); med. large (16-16½);
large (17-17½). *State size.* Shpg. wt. ea. 1 lb. 7 oz.

[H] **California-made**—you know it's a style leader!
All-rayon, superbly tailored—high-lighted with
2-tone zipper front, 2 diagonal pockets, stitchless
collar. Single button cuffs. Hand wash . . . max.
3% fabric shrinkage. *State size above.* Boxed.
33 E 739—Maroon front and gray background
33 E 740—Beige front, luggage brown ground
33 E 741—Blue front and gray background
Each . . . . $4.88   2 for $9.50

**Diagonal-slash zipper; hand
washable rayon gabardine** $4.88 Each

[J] All eyes slant toward you when you wear this
California-made "style-blazer"—it angles for
compliments! Bold, diagonal-slash zipper front
. . . good quality, wrinkle-scorning, all-rayon gabardine. Max. 3% fabric shrinkage. Stitchless
collar. Pearl type gripper fastener on cuffs and
on single flap pocket. Boxed. *State size above.*
33 E 735—Tan 33 E 736—Gray 33 E 737—Brown
33 E 738—Blue. Each . . . . . $4.88   2 for $9.50

ALL **PAGE 333 . . MEN'S SPORT SHIRTS**

115

Outerwear

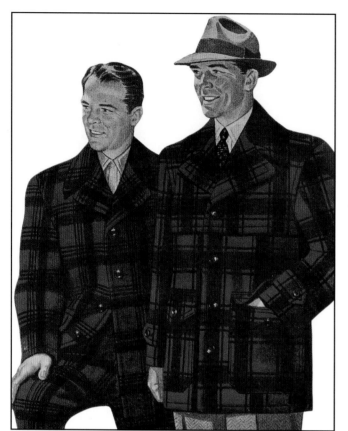

Hercules double-back stag coats, red and black plaid, 50% pure virgin wool, 50% tough reused wool. $9-12. [$10-20] Matching breeches of same material, $6. [$5-10] *Fall/winter 1946-1947*

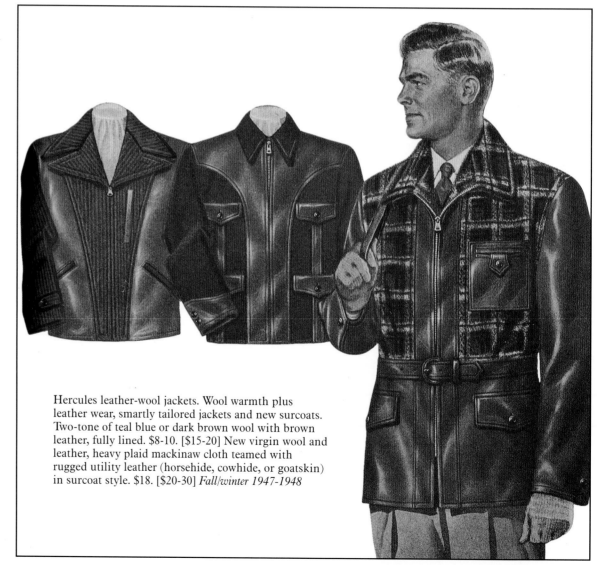

Hercules leather-wool jackets. Wool warmth plus leather wear, smartly tailored jackets and new surcoats. Two-tone of teal blue or dark brown wool with brown leather, fully lined. $8-10. [$15-20] New virgin wool and leather, heavy plaid mackinaw cloth teamed with rugged utility leather (horsehide, cowhide, or goatskin) in surcoat style. $18. [$20-30] *Fall/winter 1947-1948*

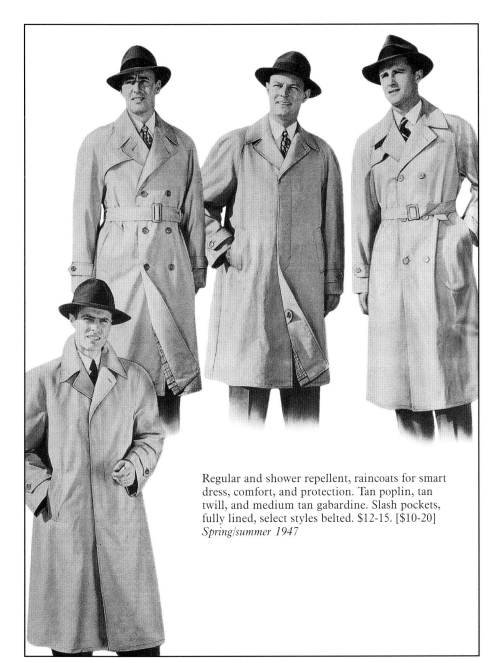

Regular and shower repellent, raincoats for smart dress, comfort, and protection. Tan poplin, tan twill, and medium tan gabardine. Slash pockets, fully lined, select styles belted. $12-15. [$10-20] *Spring/summer 1947*

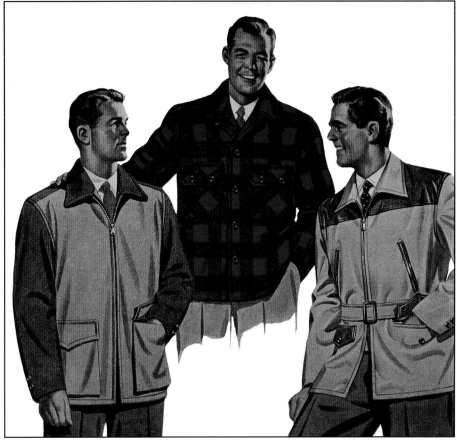

Jackets for spring…wool, leather, or cotton, twenty-five to thirty-inch lengths. Casual parksuede surcoat, in camel tan and cocoa brown. New wool plaid jacket, in red and black or white and black. Leather trimmed surcoat, in tan poplin with brown capeskin trim. $10-14. [$10-20] *Spring/summer 1947*

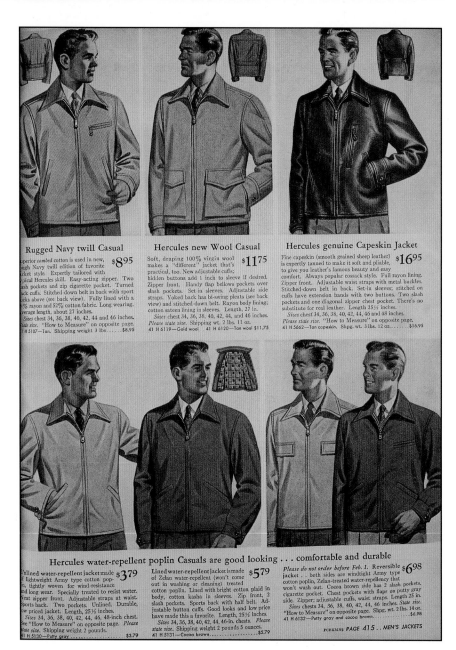

Rugged Navy twill Casual $8⁹⁵

superior *combed* cotton is used in new, rugh Navy twill edition of favorite jacket style. Expertly tailored with typical Hercules skill. Easy-acting zipper. Two slash pockets and zip cigarette pocket. Turned back cuffs. Stitched-down belt in back with sport tucks above (see back view). Fully lined with a 48% rayon and 52% cotton fabric. Long wearing, average length, about 27 inches.
State size. "How to Measure" on opposite page.
41 H 5107—Tan. Shipping weight 3 lbs......$8.95

Hercules new Wool Casual $11⁷⁵

Soft, draping 100% virgin wool makes a "different" jacket that's practical, too. New adjustable cuffs: hidden buttons add 1 inch to sleeve if desired. Zipper front. Handy flap bellows pockets over slash pockets. Set-in sleeves. Adjustable side straps. Yoked back has bi-swing pleats (see back view) and stitched-down belt. Rayon body lining; cotton sateen lining in sleeves. Length, 27 in.
Sizes chest 34, 36, 38, 40, 42, 44, and 46 inches. *Please state size.* Shipping wt. 2 lbs. 11 oz.
41 H 6119—Gold wool   41 H 6120—Tan wool $11.75

Hercules genuine Capeskin Jacket $16⁹⁵

Fine capeskin (smooth grained sheep leather) is expertly tanned to make it soft and pliable, to give you leather's famous beauty and easy comfort. Always popular cossack style. Full rayon lining. Zipper front. Adjustable waist straps with metal buckles. Stitched-down belt in back. Set-in sleeves; stitched on cuffs have extension bands with two buttons. Two slash pockets and one diagonal zipper chest pocket. There's no substitute for real leather. Length 25½ inches.
Sizes chest 34, 36, 38, 40, 42, 44, 46 and 48 inches.
Please state size. "How to Measure" on opposite page.
41 H 5662—Tan capeskin. Shpg. wt. 3 lbs. 12 oz........$16.95

Hercules water-repellent poplin Casuals are good looking . . . comfortable and durable

Unlined water-repellent jacket made $3⁷⁹ of lightweight Army type cotton poplin, tightly woven for wind-resistance and long wear. Specially treated to resist water. Neat zipper front. Adjustable straps at waist. Sports back. Two pockets. Unlined. Durable, low priced jacket. Length, 25¼ inches.
Sizes 34, 36, 38, 40, 42, 44, 46, 48-inch chest.
See "How to Measure" on opposite page. *Please state size.* Shipping weight 2 pounds.
41 H 5130—Putty gray..........$3.79

Lined water-repellent jacket is made $5⁷⁹ of Zelan water-repellent (won't come out in washing or cleaning) treated cotton poplin. Lined with bright cotton plaid in body, cotton kasha in sleeves. Zip front, 2 slash pockets. Sports back with half belt. Adjustable button cuffs. Good looks and low price have made this a favorite. Length, 25¼ inches.
Sizes 34, 36, 38, 40, 42, 44, 46-in. chests. *Please state size.* Shipping weight 2 pounds 5 ounces.
41 H 5131—Cocoa brown...........$5.79

Please do not order before Feb. 1. Reversible $6⁹⁸ jacket . . both sides are windtight Army type cotton poplin, Zelan-treated water-repellency that won't wash out. Cocoa brown side has 2 slash pockets, cigarette pocket. Chest pockets with flaps on putty gray side. Zipper; adjustable cuffs, waist straps. Length 25 in.
Sizes chests 34, 36, 38, 40, 42, 44, 46 inches. *State size.* "How to Measure" on opposite page. Shpg. wt. 2 lbs. 14 oz.
41 H 6132—Putty gray and cocoa brown...........$6.98

PCBKMN∂ PAGE 415 .. MEN'S JACKETS

Rugged navy twill casual, wool casual, capeskin jacket, or water-repellent poplin casuals…comfortable and durable, great for the warmer months. $4-16. [$10-15] *Spring/summer 1947*

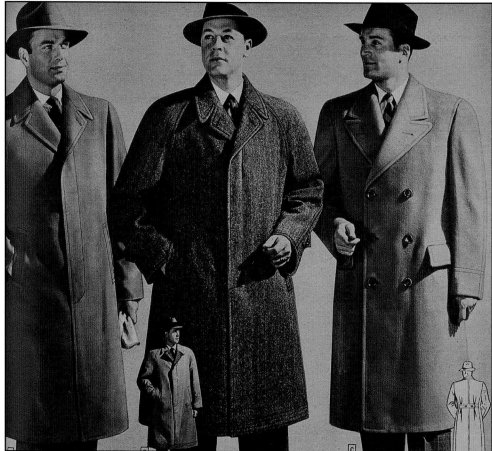

Topcoats…Fashion Tailored gabardine and 100% all wool in smart, popular types…built for longer wear, cut for greater comfort. Water repellent style in grayish tan or dark tan gabardine, reversible in blue or brown, or all wool polo coat in camel. $16-30. [$15-20] *Fall/winter 1948*

118

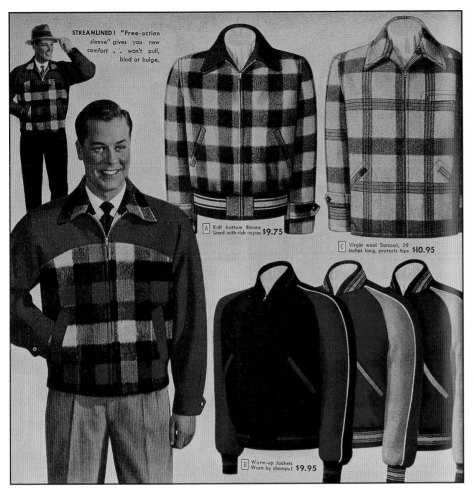

STREAMLINED! "Free-action sleeve" gives you new comfort . . . won't pull, bind or bulge.

A   Knit bottom Blouse Lined with rich rayon **$9.75**

C   Virgin wool Surcoat, 29 inches long, protects hips **$10.95**

B   Warm-up Jackets Worn by champs! **$9.95**

100% wool Action-Jacket, in rust brown or sport blue with buffalo plaid front. Knit bottom virgin wool jacket, smart plaid front and sleeves, rich solid tone collar and back, snug fitting bottom, brown and white. Athletic style warm-up jacket, sparkling colors in warm wool, body lined with fancy cotton flannel, in royal and scarlet, scarlet and gray, or green and gray. 100% virgin wool plaid surcoat, so warm, needs no lining, in windowpane plaid. $10-13. [$10-20] *Fall/winter 1948*

Choice leathers…fully lined zip-fronts. Brown suede, tan capeskin, or black horsehide. Leather blouse, in Cossack or aviator style. $15-20. [$20-30] *Fall/winter 1948*

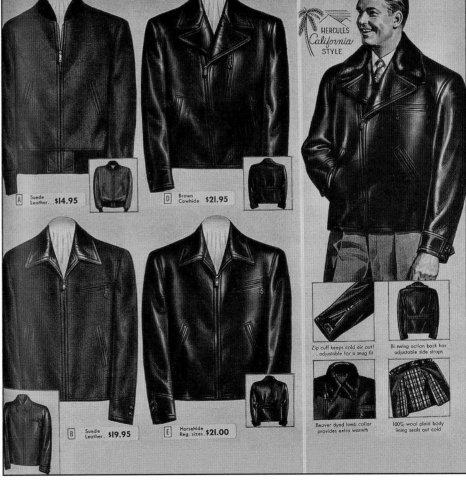

HERCULES California STYLE

A   Suede Leather.. **$14.95**

D   Brown Cowhide **$21.95**

B   Suede Leather. **$19.95**

E   Horsehide Reg. sizes **$21.00**

Zip cuff keeps cold air out! . . . adjustable for a snug fit

Bi-swing action back has adjustable side straps

Beaver dyed lamb collar provides extra warmth

100% wool plaid body lining seals out cold

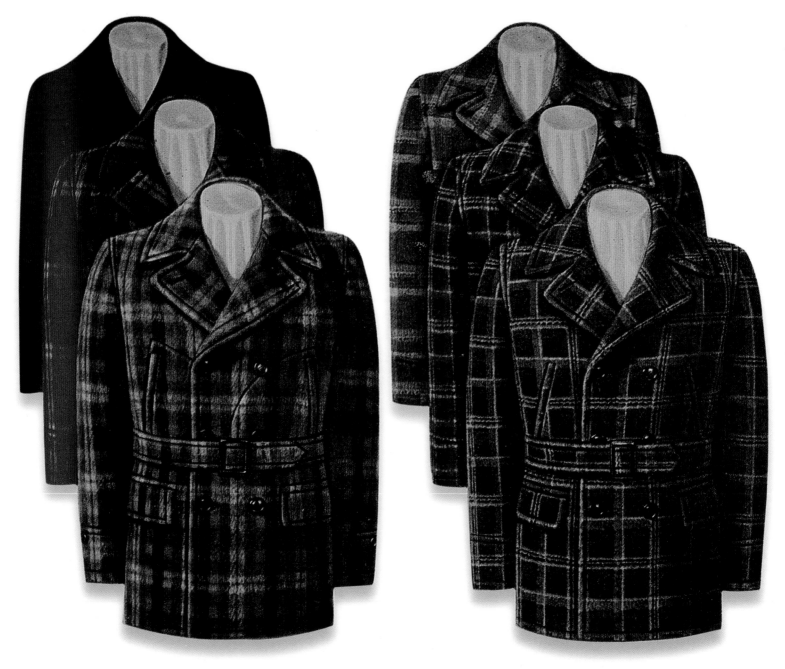

All wool Mackinaws, unlined or warmly lined, wool plaids, or navy blue melton. $7, $13. Two-tone jacket and sportsman-style jacket with knit bottom, zipper-front, in navy blue melton or two-tone blue plaid. $6. [$10-20] *Fall/winter 1948*

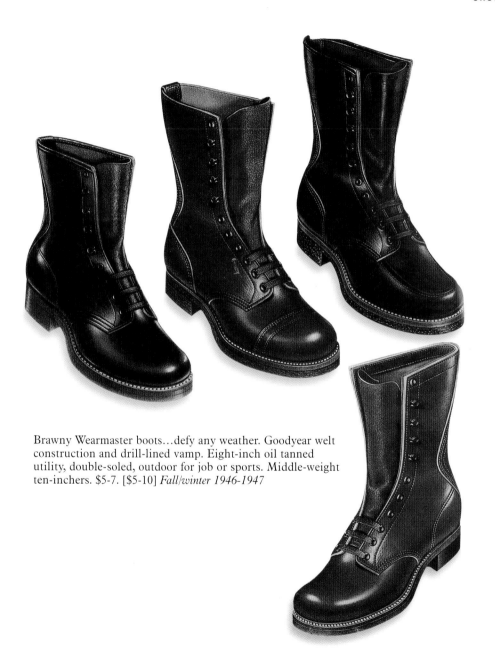

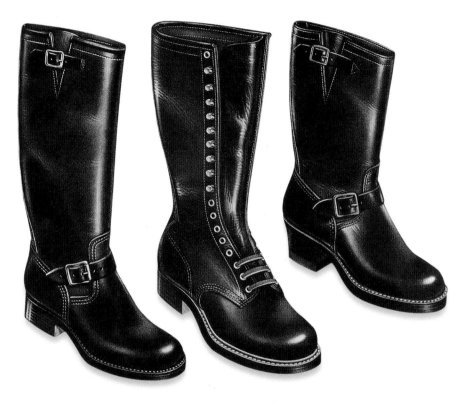

Brawny Wearmaster boots…defy any weather. Goodyear welt construction and drill-lined vamp. Eight-inch oil tanned utility, double-soled, outdoor for job or sports. Middle-weight ten-inchers. $5-7. [$5-10] *Fall/winter 1946-1947*

Seventeen-inch Engineers' boots, oil tanned, black. Sixteen-inch lace-up boot, or eleven-inch Engineer Woodsman-heel boot, double oil tanned, oak leather midsole. $10-17. [$10-20] *Spring/summer 1947*

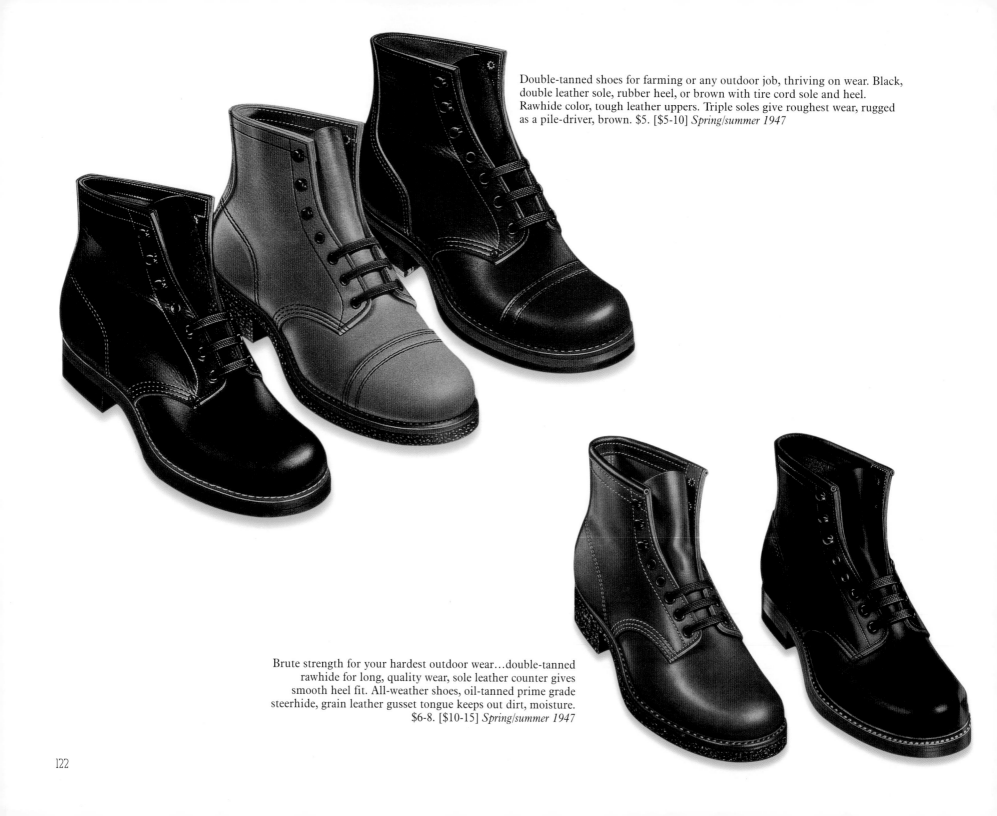

Double-tanned shoes for farming or any outdoor job, thriving on wear. Black, double leather sole, rubber heel, or brown with tire cord sole and heel. Rawhide color, tough leather uppers. Triple soles give roughest wear, rugged as a pile-driver, brown. $5. [$5-10] *Spring/summer 1947*

Brute strength for your hardest outdoor wear…double-tanned rawhide for long, quality wear, sole leather counter gives smooth heel fit. All-weather shoes, oil-tanned prime grade steerhide, grain leather gusset tongue keeps out dirt, moisture. $6-8. [$10-15] *Spring/summer 1947*

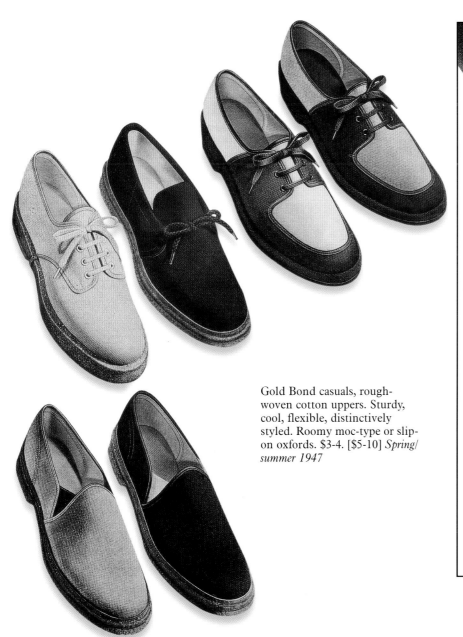

Gold Bond casuals, rough-woven cotton uppers. Sturdy, cool, flexible, distinctively styled. Roomy moc-type or slip-on oxfords. $3-4. [$5-10] *Spring/summer 1947*

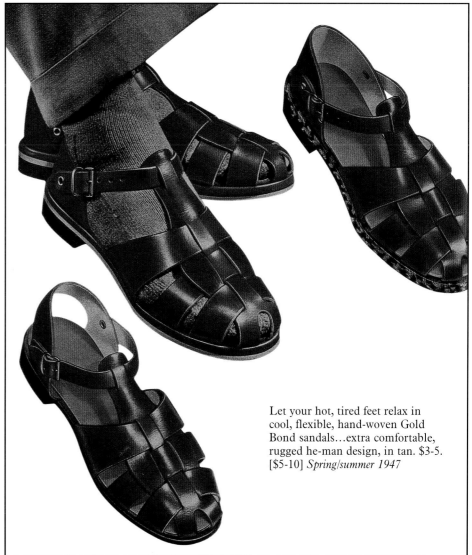

Let your hot, tired feet relax in cool, flexible, hand-woven Gold Bond sandals…extra comfortable, rugged he-man design, in tan. $3-5. [$5-10] *Spring/summer 1947*

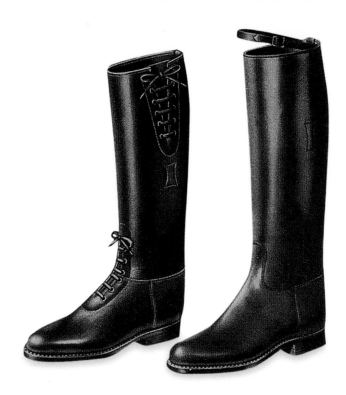

Gold Bond Cowboy boots, genuine Texas-made, fine grain leathers, pegged shanks. Wearmaster field and riding boots…made by Kirkendall. Grain leather with soft leather lining, in brown with tan vamp, solid brown, or black. $14-20. [$10-20] *Fall/winter 1948*

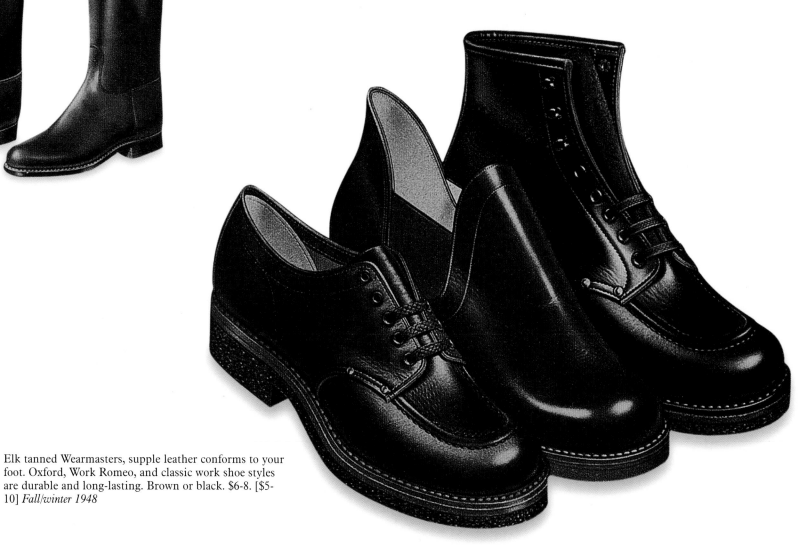

Elk tanned Wearmasters, supple leather conforms to your foot. Oxford, Work Romeo, and classic work shoe styles are durable and long-lasting. Brown or black. $6-8. [$5-10] *Fall/winter 1948*

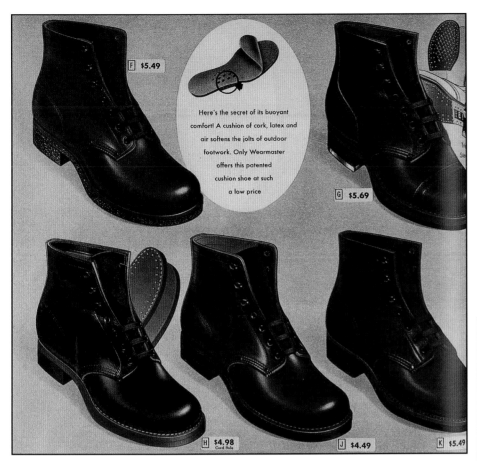

Patented cushion insole, triple sole with steel rim heel, thrifty grain leather shoe. Goodyear welt construction, flexible, yet shape- retaining. Brown or black leather. $5-6. [$5-10] *Fall/winter 1948*

Top quality rubber Wearmasters, super-strong and long-wearing for the roughest, wettest jobs. Tough white rubber soles. Different heights. $3-6. [$5-10] *Fall/winter 1948*

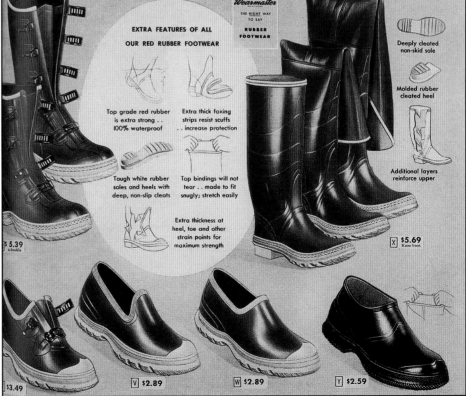

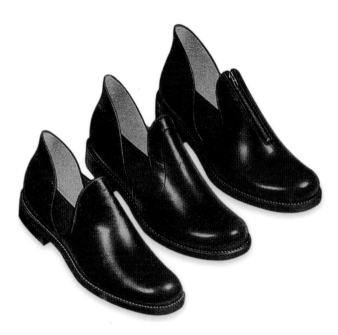

Men's and boys' Romeos, your favorite "ho-hum-ers"…soft kidskin uppers, leather soles. Three qualities. Camp-mocs, husky leather uppers, for relaxing indoors or out. Genuine leather Gold Bond slippers, to ease your yawning hours. $3-5. [$5-10] *Fall/winter 1948*

Cushioned Gold Bonds, scoop styling. A success in any setting…business or fun. Cord-stitched trim, plain toe, scotch grain leather, or Algonquin moc-styles, in brown, black, and dark wine-tone. $11. [$5-10] *Fall/winter 1948*

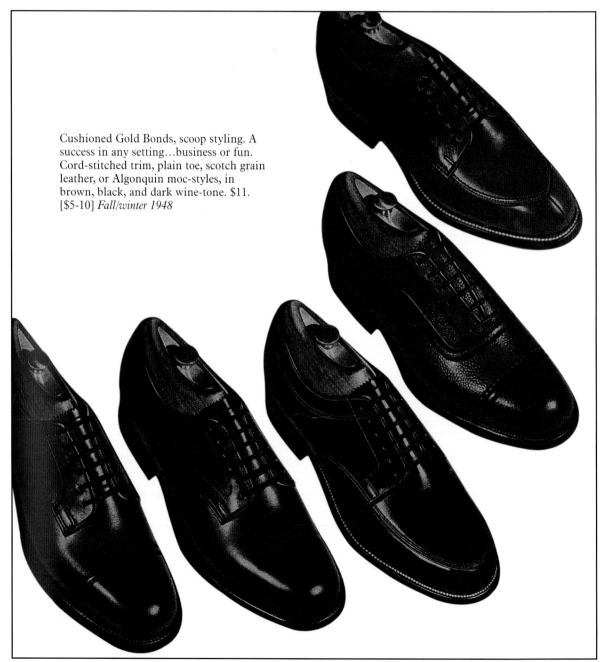

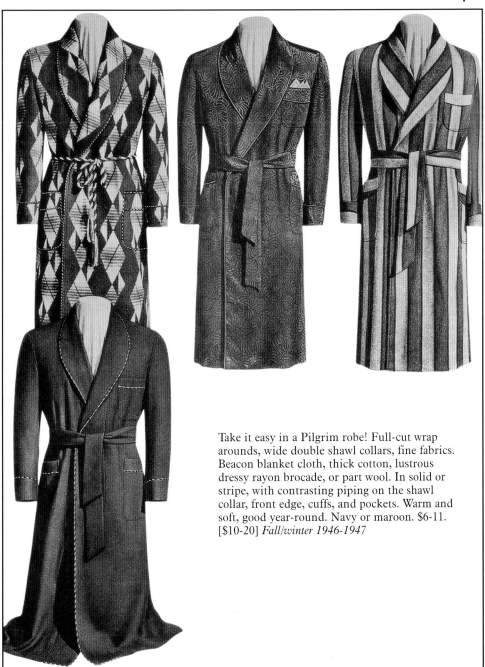

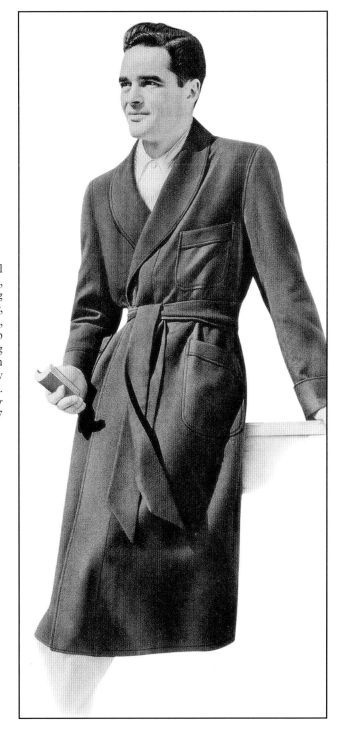

Take it easy in a Pilgrim robe! Full-cut wrap arounds, wide double shawl collars, fine fabrics. Beacon blanket cloth, thick cotton, lustrous dressy rayon brocade, or part wool. In solid or stripe, with contrasting piping on the shawl collar, front edge, cuffs, and pockets. Warm and soft, good year-round. Navy or maroon. $6-11. [$10-20] *Fall/winter 1946-1947*

100% virgin wool flannel robe, smooth-fitting double shawl collar, well cut shoulders, matching non-slip sash, contrasting cord piping, medium weight fabric. Navy or maroon. $11-14. [$10-20] *Fall/winter 1946-1947*

127

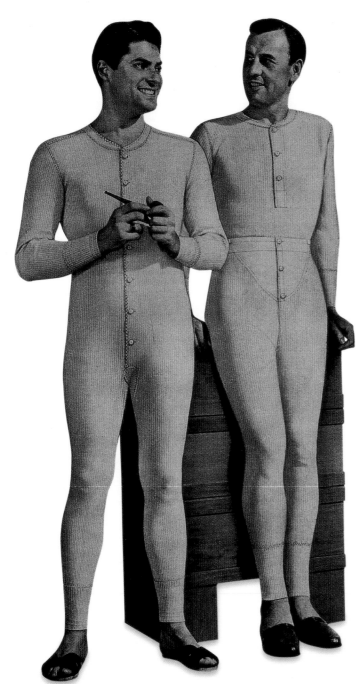

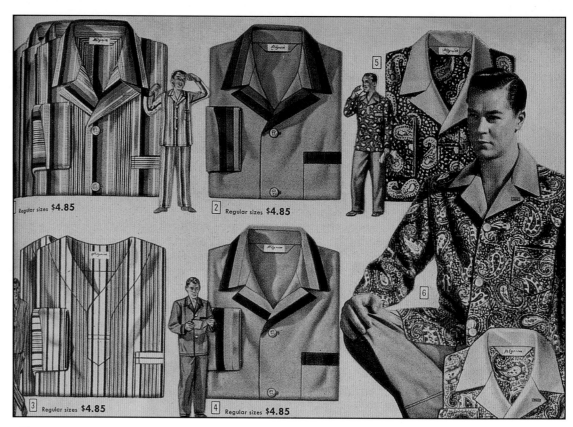

Fine quality smooth cotton broadcloth or Sanforized pajamas. Full-cut and roomy for restful sleep, drawstring waistband or trouser-type snap fly. Striped, two-tone trim, or paisley printed. $4-5. [$5-10] *Fall/winter 1948*

Union suits, shirts, and drawers. Rib knit, warm, heavy, with the kind of comfort, wear, and Pilgrim reliability outdoor men demand. Cream or gray. $1-2. [$3-5] *Spring/summer 1947*

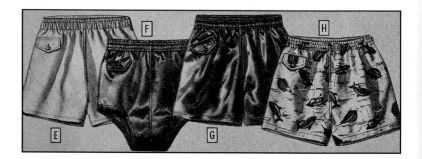

Cotton twill swim trunks. Rayon satin, shiny side out, boxer style, lastex yarn. Rayon satin swim trunks, speed style, smooth fit. Tan, blue, maize (yellow), or maroon, with multicolored print. $1-4. [$5-10] *Spring/summer 1949*

Dress Wear

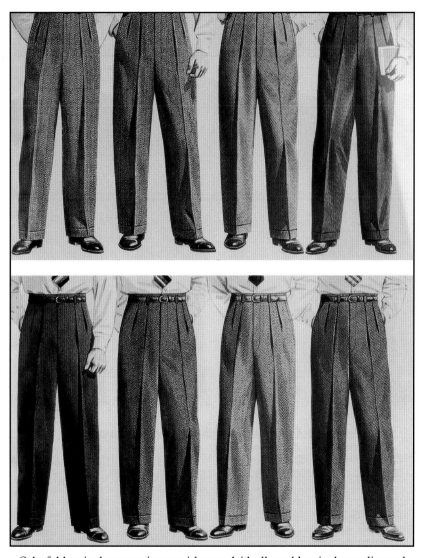

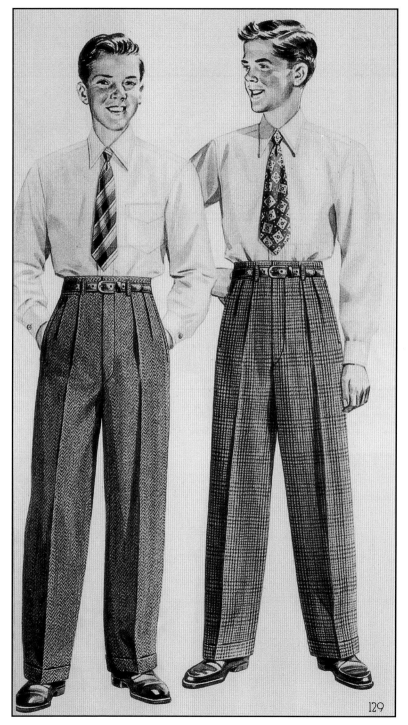

Colorful herringbone cassimere with overplaid, all wool herringbone, diagonal twill weave, fine quality gabardine with zipper front, serviceable part wool cheviot, or narrow herringbone weave part wool cassimere styles…in medium brown, medium blue, or dark brown. All Fraternity Prep quality and comfort. $4-5. [$5-10] *Fall/winter 1946-1947*

Dress slacks for young men…100% new wool, zipper-front, hard wearing, shape-retaining fabrics, with Fraternity Prep quality tailoring. Deluxe quality herringbone, in blue or brown, and colorful glen plaid, in medium blue or brown. $4-6. [$5-10] *Fall/winter 1946-1947*

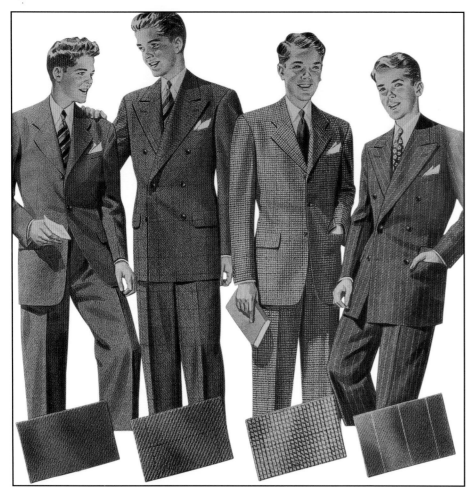

Fraternity Prep fall suits, styled in the spirit of youth. Rich, 100% virgin wools. Distinctive diagonal weave, drape style, all wool tweed-like suiting, or chalk stripe. All trim fitting trousers have pleats, cuffs, and dropped belt loops. Medium blue, medium brown, or dark tan. $16-18. [$10-20] *Fall/winter 1946-1947*

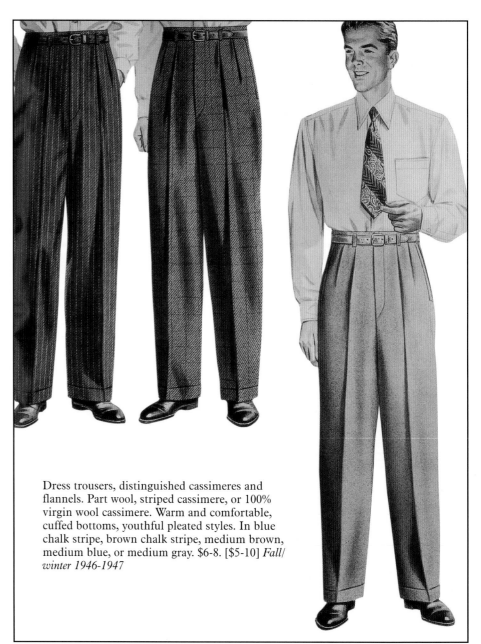

Dress trousers, distinguished cassimeres and flannels. Part wool, striped cassimere, or 100% virgin wool cassimere. Warm and comfortable, cuffed bottoms, youthful pleated styles. In blue chalk stripe, brown chalk stripe, medium brown, medium blue, or medium gray. $6-8. [$5-10] *Fall/winter 1946-1947*

Casual

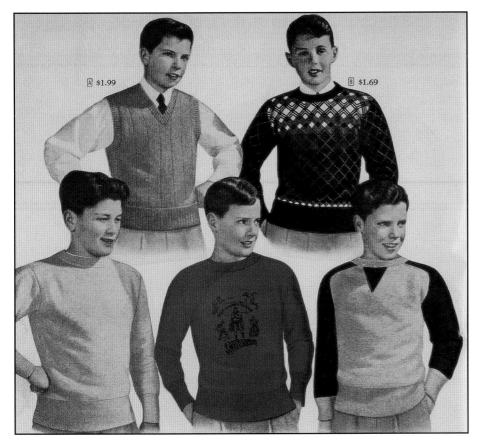

Pullovers and sweatshirts every active fellow needs for work and play. All wool sleeveless sweater, good-looking cotton pullover, warm flat knit cotton sweatshirt, new "Superman" sweatshirt, and full freedom sleeve sweatshirt. $1-2. [$5-10] *Fall/winter 1946-1947*

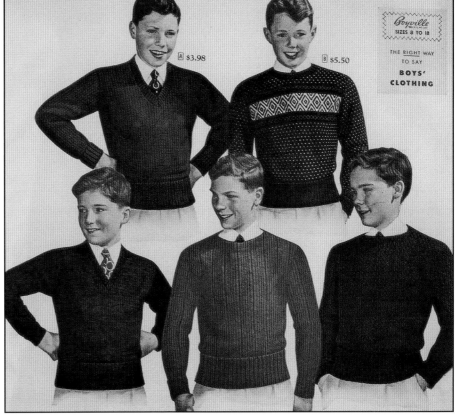

Colorful pullovers by Boyville…he'll wear them for school and dress. 100% all wool worsted, panel rib knit or heavy shaker pullover. Swiss-like popular ski-type pattern or solids. Medium brown, camel tan, light blue, maroon, or navy blue. $1-4. [$5-10] *Fall/winter 1946-1947*

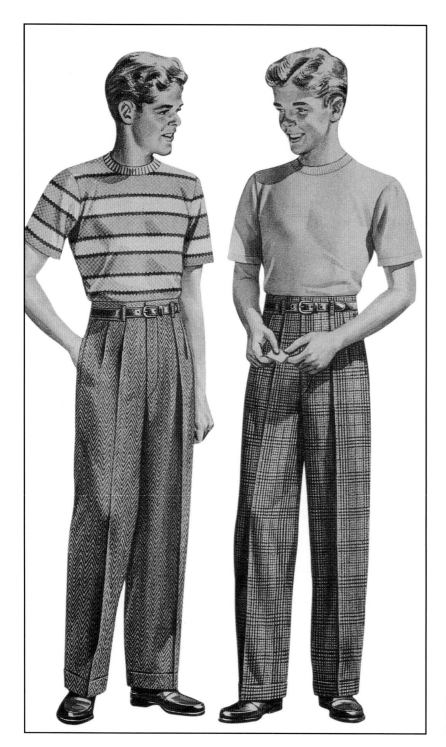

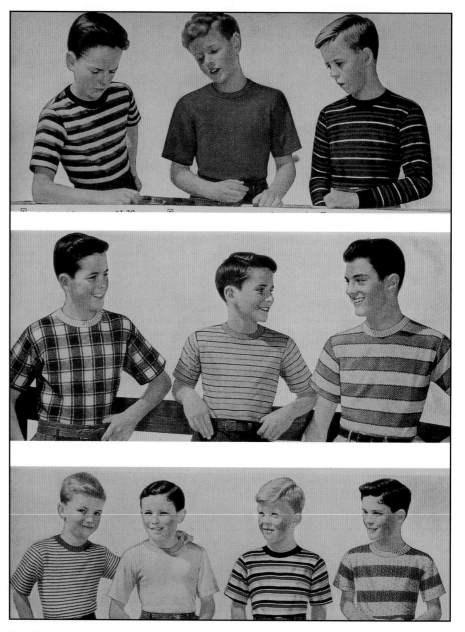

Boyville cotton tee shirts, neat looking, fellows want them by the dozen! Two-ply combed cotton, smart carded knit, plaid, striped, or string knit shirts. Club stripes, fine combed cotton, and heavy string knit styles, in bold, exciting colors. $1-2. [$5-10] *Spring/summer 1947*

Smart zipper-front slacks, 100% new wool. Fine quality herringbone, rich colorful glen plaid. Smooth drape, deep roomy pockets, Fraternity Prep charm. $6. [$5-10] String knit shirt in novelty pattern, or cool cotton knit shirt in gay plain colors. $1-2. [$5-10] *Spring/summer 1947*

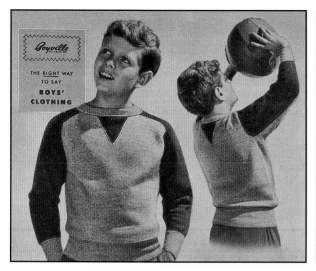

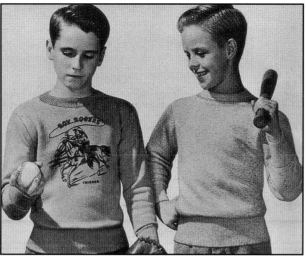

All purpose sweatshirts, designed for active boys' sports, full-cut for comfort. Heavyweight flat knit cotton, thick cotton fleecing inside. Oxford gray with royal trim. "Roy Rogers" sweatshirt, popular cowboy theme, and good quality sweatshirt, sturdy flat knit cotton, double ribbed cuffs, neck, and bottom fit snugly. Medium blue, red, or silver gray. $1-2. [$5-10] *Spring/summer 1947*

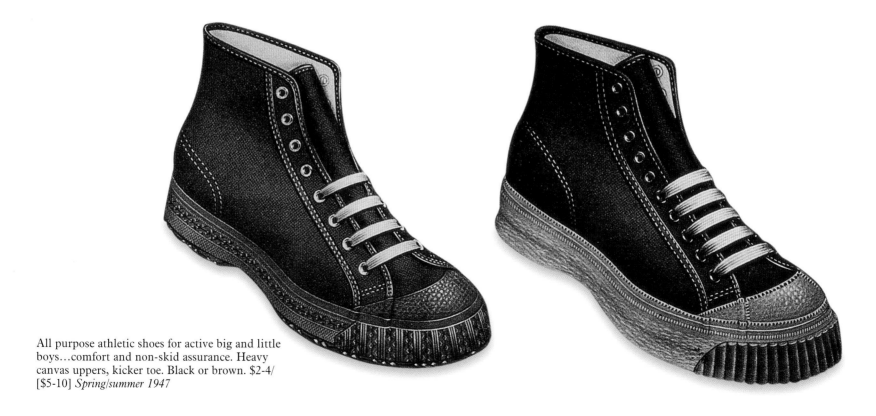

All purpose athletic shoes for active big and little boys…comfort and non-skid assurance. Heavy canvas uppers, kicker toe. Black or brown. $2-4/ [$5-10] *Spring/summer 1947*

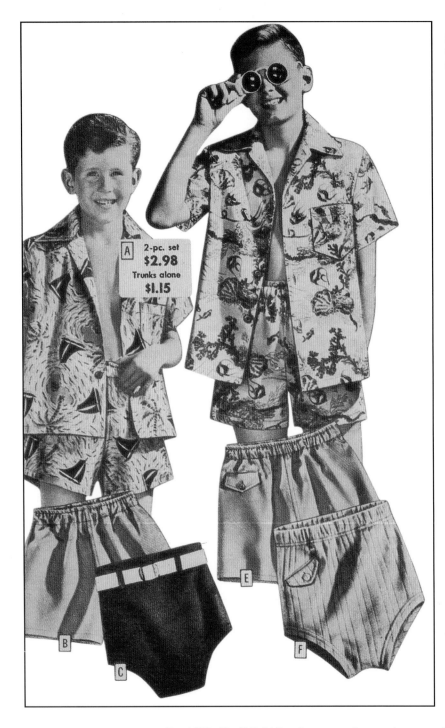

A | 2-pc. set
$2.98
Trunks alone
$1.15

Swimwear, smartly styled in the California manner. Trunks and festive summer shorts, Sanforized vat-dyed cotton or 100% wool worsted, boxer style swim shorts. Navy, maroon, tan, or medium blue combinations. $1-4. [5-10] *Spring/summer 1949*

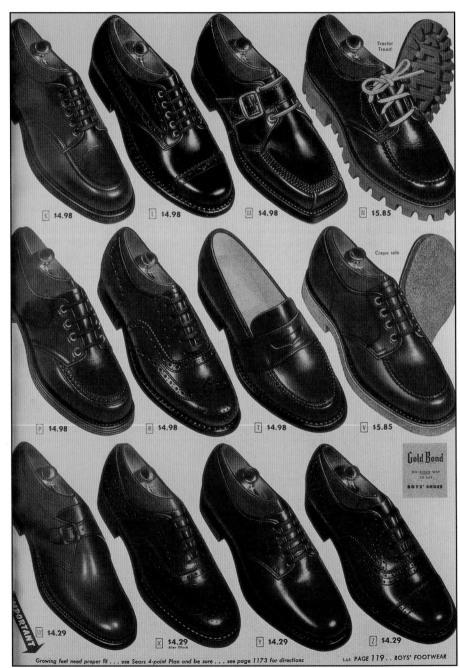

Boys' "He-Man" Gold Bonds, snappy dress styles, room for growth. Casual, oxford, and moc-style shoes, in brown leather or wine-tone. Great for school or dates. $4-6. [$10-15] *Spring/summer 1949*

134

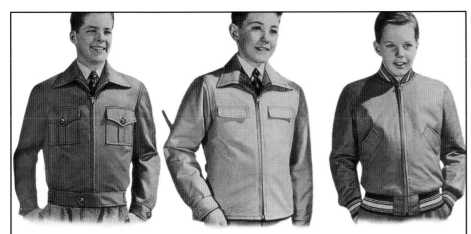

Heavy poplin battle-style jacket, double duty reversible jacket. All wool pile lined poplin, capeskin leather and melton cloth, brown melton, or all wool melton. In navy, cocoa brown, or dark brown. $4-9. [$10-15] *Fall/winter 1946-1947*

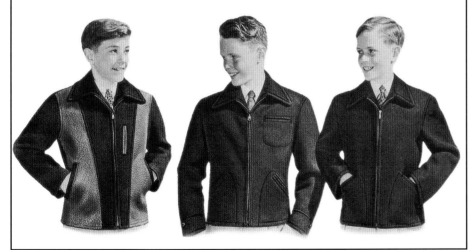

All weather hats and caps…Boyville-made, with all the rugged style and snug warmth fellows want. $1-2. [$5-10] *Fall/winter 1946-1947*

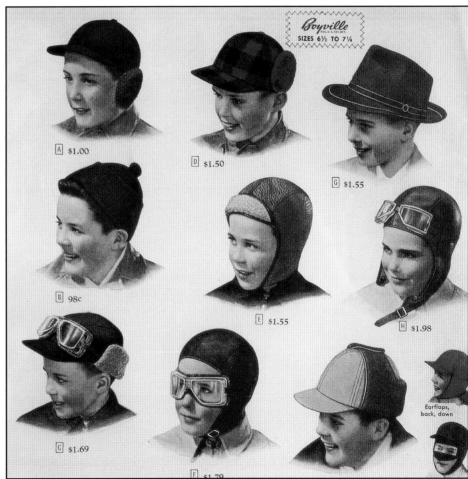

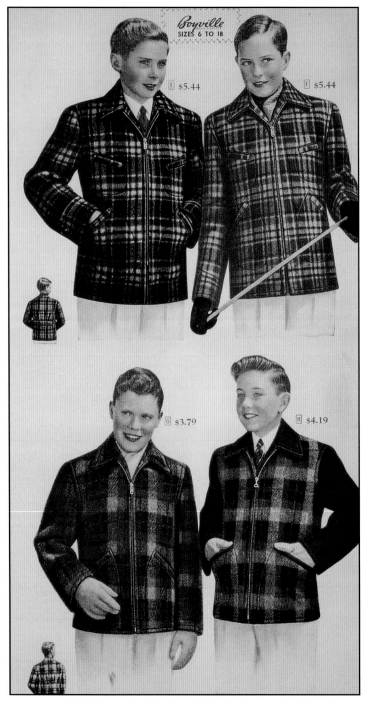

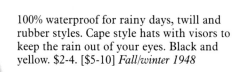

100% virgin wool winter fleece "shirt-tail" length jackets. Smart patterns, zipper-fronts. Blue, brown two-tone, maroon, or blue plaid. $4-6. [$10-15] *Fall/winter 1946-1947*

100% waterproof for rainy days, twill and rubber styles. Cape style hats with visors to keep the rain out of your eyes. Black and yellow. $2-4. [$5-10] *Fall/winter 1948*

Sheepskin or pile-lined all-weather coats, husky smartness and deep, dependable warmth to make winter fun! Moleskin with rich lambskin shawl collar, double-breasted corduroy, or gabardine with lambskin collar. $10-14. [$10-15] *Fall/winter 1948*

CHILDREN'S FASHIONS

Dresses and Suits

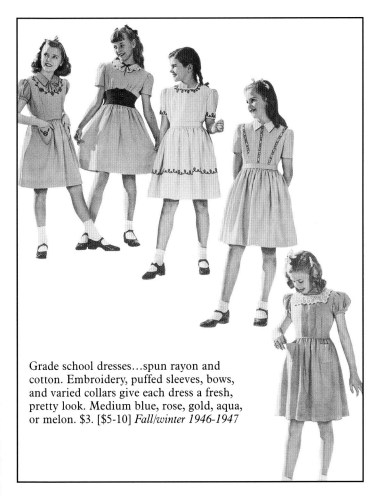

Grade school dresses...spun rayon and cotton. Embroidery, puffed sleeves, bows, and varied collars give each dress a fresh, pretty look. Medium blue, rose, gold, aqua, or melon. $3. [$5-10] *Fall/winter 1946-1947*

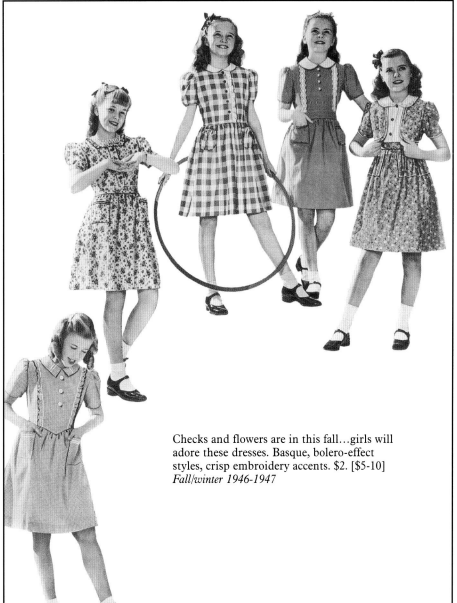

Checks and flowers are in this fall...girls will adore these dresses. Basque, bolero-effect styles, crisp embroidery accents. $2. [$5-10] *Fall/winter 1946-1947*

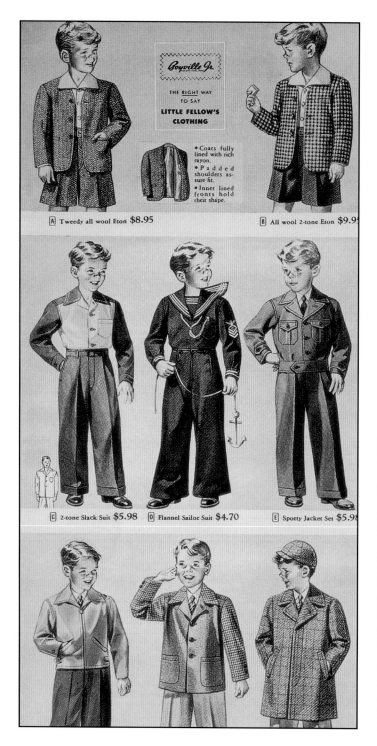

Boyville Jr.

THE RIGHT WAY
TO SAY
LITTLE FELLOW'S
CLOTHING

• Coats fully lined with rich rayon.
• Padded shoulders assure fit.
• Inner lined fronts hold their shape.

[A] Tweedy all wool Eton $8.95

[B] All wool 2-tone Eton $9.95

[C] 2-tone Slack Suit $5.98

[D] Flannel Sailor Suit $4.70

[E] Sporty Jacket Set $5.98

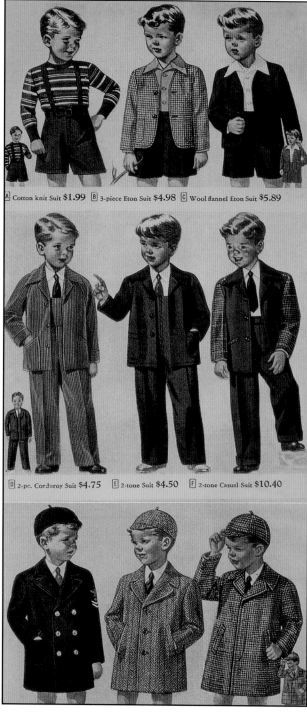

[A] Cotton knit Suit $1.99

[B] 3-piece Eton Suit $4.98

[C] Wool flannel Eton Suit $5.89

[D] 2-pc. Corduroy Suit $4.75

[E] 2-tone Suit $4.50

[F] 2-tone Casual Suit $10.40

LEFT · Two-tone brown and tan cotton gabardine slack suit. Tan front, dark brown back, sleeves, and collar. Pleated longies. Navy blue sailor suit in part wool flannel, with firmly anchored buttons. Sanforized cotton gabardine twill jacket and pleated longies. $5-6. [$10-15] *Spring/summer 1947*

RIGHT · Eton suits for the little ones…Boyville Jr. makes a rugged, hard wearing outfit. Shortie and longie styles, in rich wool flannel, pinwale corduroy, or cotton gabardine. Navy, medium blue, or brown. $2-6. [$5-10] *Spring/summer 1947*

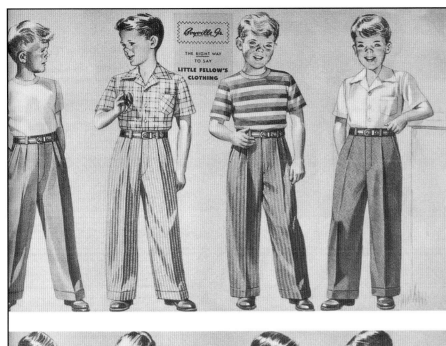

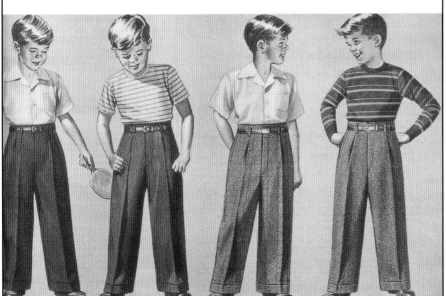

Year-round longies, styles to please little guys. Cotton poplin, crisp Sanforized seersucker, herringbone, or gabardine twill, in medium blue or brown. Navy blue part wool cheviot, blue or brown blended twill weave gabardine, rich wool and rayon blend in smooth finish cassimere, or all wool herringbone weave. All with cuffed bottoms and dropped belt loops. $1-4. [$5-10] *Spring/summer 1947*

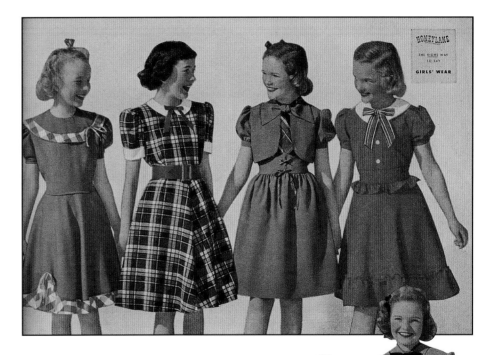

Honeylane fashions, swirl-skirt dresses. Spun rayon cape collar dress, blue with red check or green with green check. Peter Pan collar and big, bold, multicolor plaid. Cute bolero-effect in full-skirted labtex rayon with plaid taffeta and wonderful lacing, in Copen blue or Kelly green. Rayon ruffler has a sparkling white collar and rayon taffeta bow, in coral or Copen. "Karoma" spun rayon dress with keyhole neckline and ruffle-shirred yoke, in aqua blue or dusty rose. Gibson girl dress, light top, dark skirt, elastic-ruffled sleeves, silver buttons, in coral and navy or aqua and navy. $4-5. [$5-10] *Fall/winter 1948*

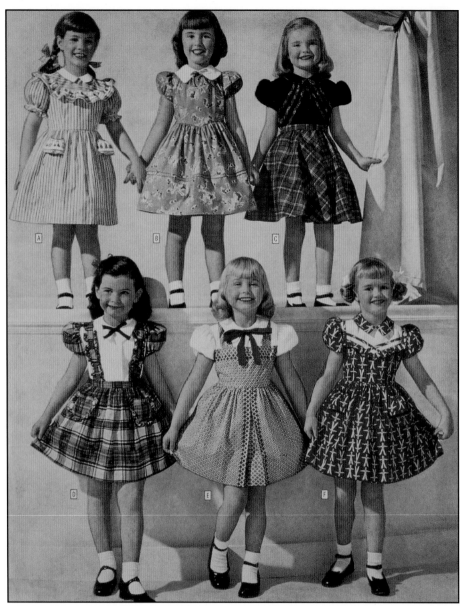

Deluxe honeysuckle cotton, hoop skirt, jumper style, and sailor boy dresses in bright colors for school or play. $3. [$5-10] *Fall/winter 1948*

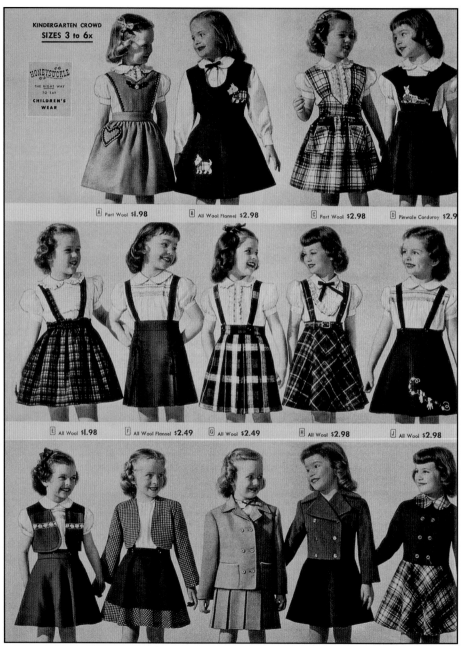

Jumpers…all little girls love them. All wool or part wool, corduroy with felt appliqués and ric-rac trim. Bright red, navy, Kelly green, or colorful plaid. All wool suspender skirts, plaids or solids, swing skirt or pleated front. Colorful plaids, reds, greens, yellows, or blues. Girls' suits with big-sister style ideas, all wool or corduroy, bolero to bellhop styles. $3-6. [$5-10] *Fall/winter 1948*

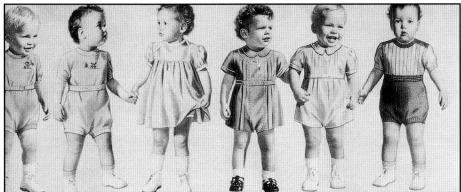

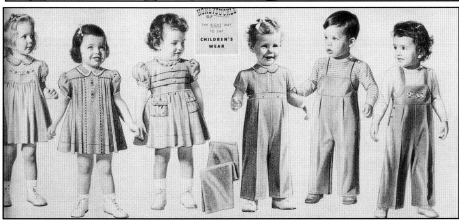

Infants' playwear, dresses and creepers in long or short styles. Yellow, blue, pink, or red. $1-2. [$5-10] *Fall/winter 1948*

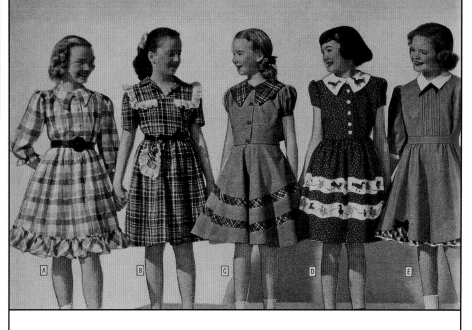

Honeylane cottons, fashionable flare-away skirts for young girls, wash and wear beautifully. Gingham plaids, cotton chambrays, ruffled yoke, appliqué trim, perky peplum, or tiered skirt styles. Bright colors for bright attitudes. $3-4. [$5-10] *Fall/winter 1948*

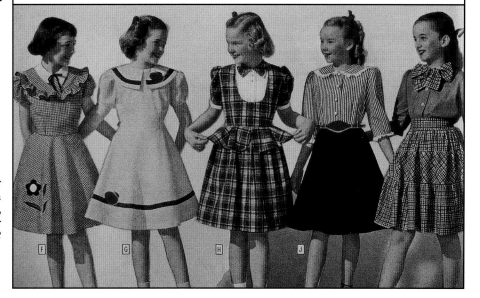

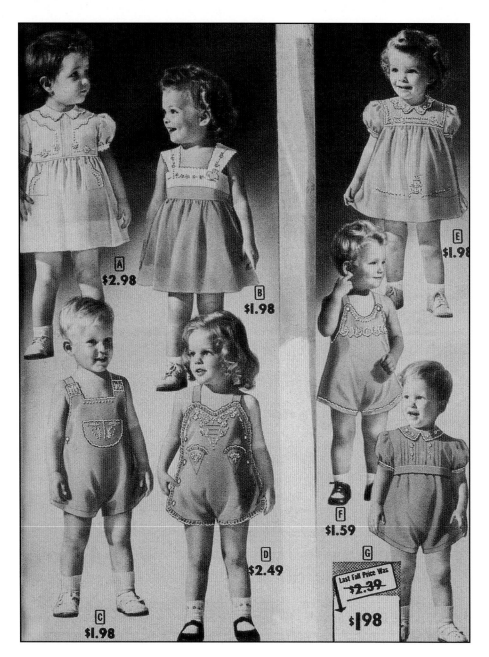

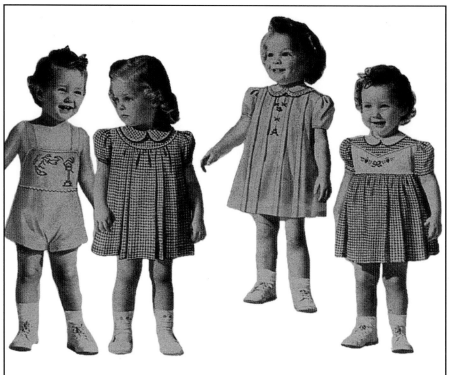

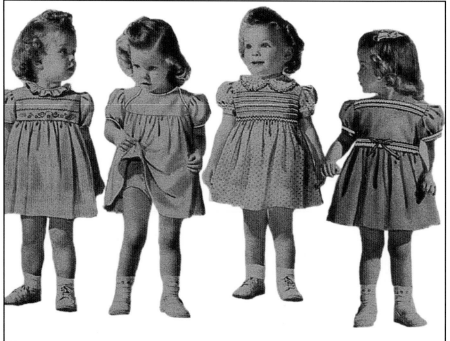

Dresses and sunsuits…combed cotton batiste and fine cotton broadcloth. Pink, yellow, blue, or white. Soft and flexible for the active baby. $2-3. [$3-5] *Spring/summer 1949*

Cotton sunsuits, broadcloth dresses with lace and embroidery. Yellow, light blue, white, pink, red. Little girls' finest cotton dresses, sheer dimity, knit cotton slip-on, dotted Swiss dress with smocked, embroidered bodice, cotton broadcloth with sheer lawn ruffles. $1-2. [$3-5] *Spring/summer 1949*

142

Playwear

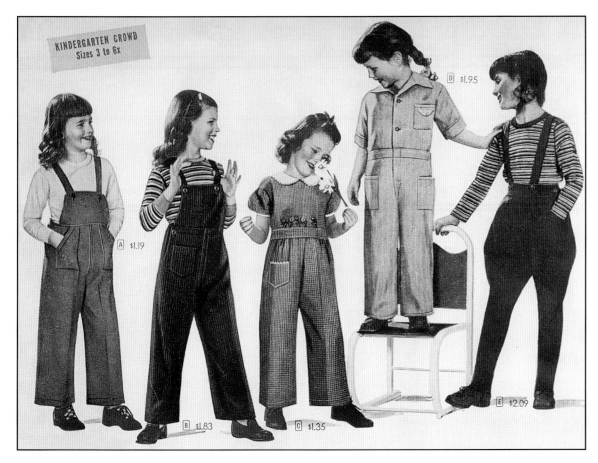

Practical playclothes…sturdy, full cut for action. Overalls, coveralls, jodhpurs, with long-sleeved sturdy knit cotton polo shirts for winter comfort. $1-2. [$5-10] *Fall/winter 1946-1947*

Neat and practical styles, shortie or longie outfits. Eton suits, sweater sets, three or four-piece playsuits, pleated cotton suiting or pinwale corduroy shorts or pants, cotton knit and chambray shirts, stripes and solids. Cadet blue, tan, teal, or dark brown. $1-5. [$5-10] *Fall/winter 1947*

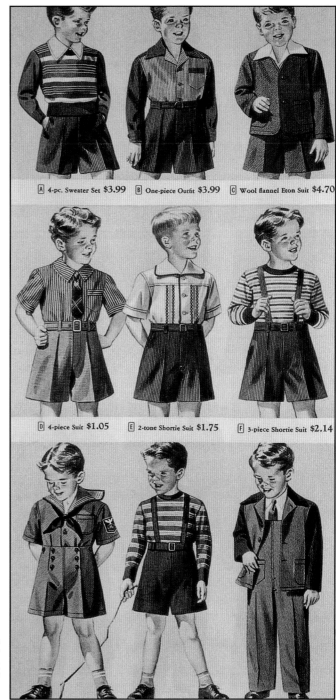

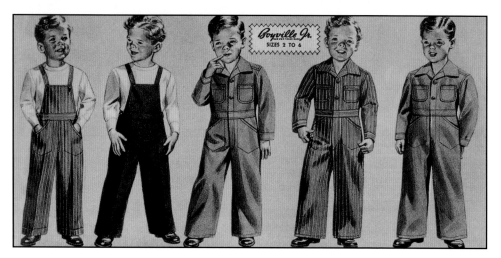

Let 'em have fun in sturdy playclothes! Sanforized striped or gabardine bib pants, cotton jean playsuit, gay corded striped playsuit, Sanforized twill playsuit. $1-2. [$5-10] *Spring/summer 1947*

Colorful multi-striped shortall in sturdy, good quality cotton. Bib top with adjustable suspenders. Sanforized cotton gabardine shortall, big patch pockets, side button opening, and yellow print styles. $2-3. [$5-10] *Spring/summer 1947*

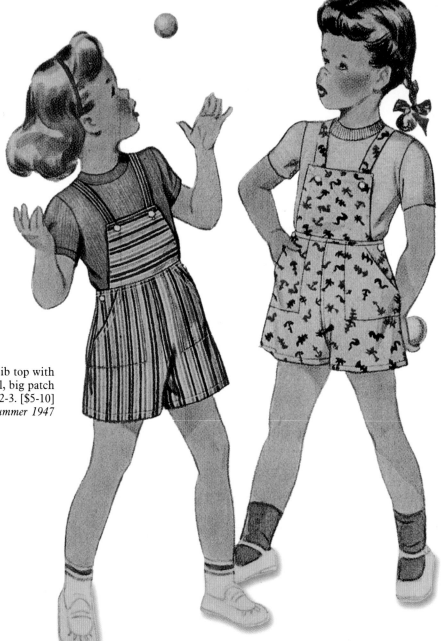

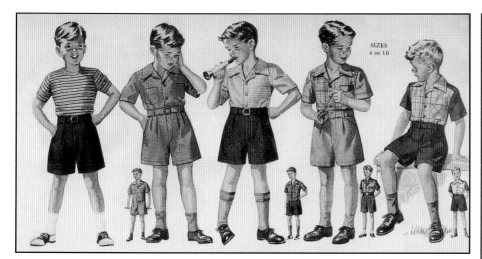

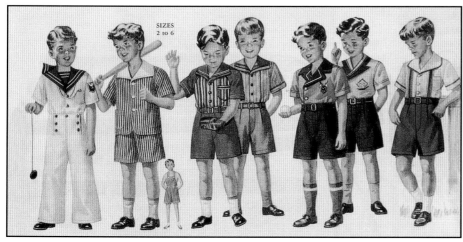

For cool, carefree summer days, Boyville Jr. shortie and play outfits. $1-3. [$5-10] *Spring/ summer 1947*

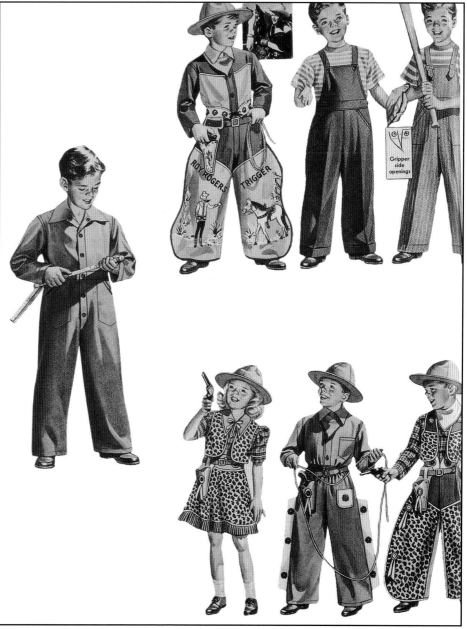

Fun in the sun, with Boyville Jr. cowboy, cowgirl, rancher, and ranger outfits, for costuming fun! Outfits come complete with lariats, holsters, and toy pistols. $2-5. [$50-75] *Spring/summer 1947*

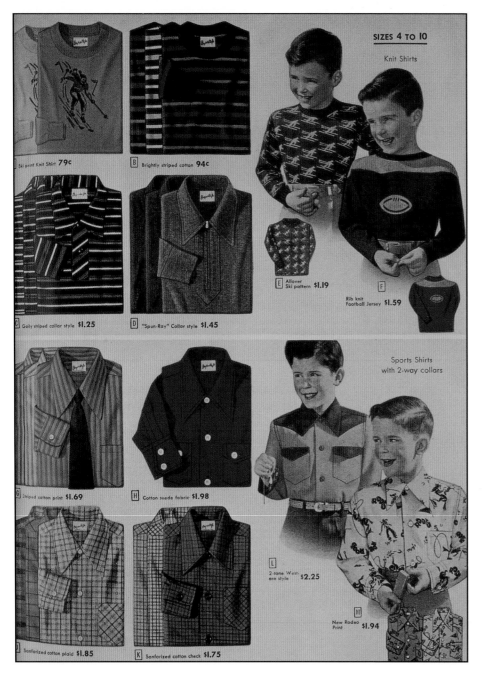

Knit and sports shirts. Durable, colorful, and extra long-wearing. Generously sized for more freedom of action. Plaids, stripes, solids, or patterns. $1-2. [$5-10] *Fall/winter 1948*

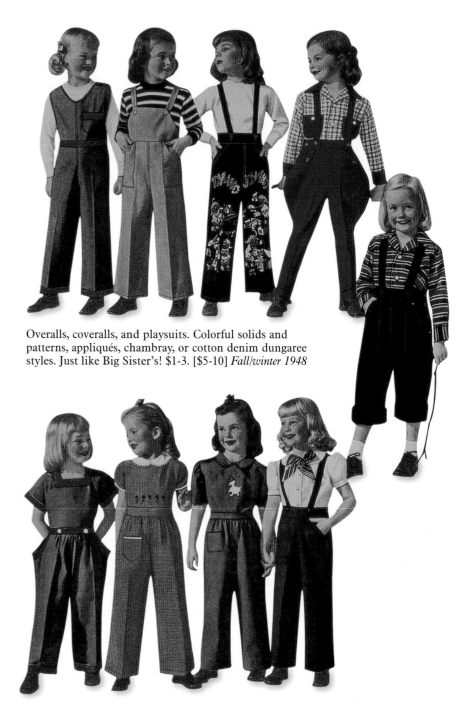

Overalls, coveralls, and playsuits. Colorful solids and patterns, appliqués, chambray, or cotton denim dungaree styles. Just like Big Sister's! $1-3. [$5-10] *Fall/winter 1948*

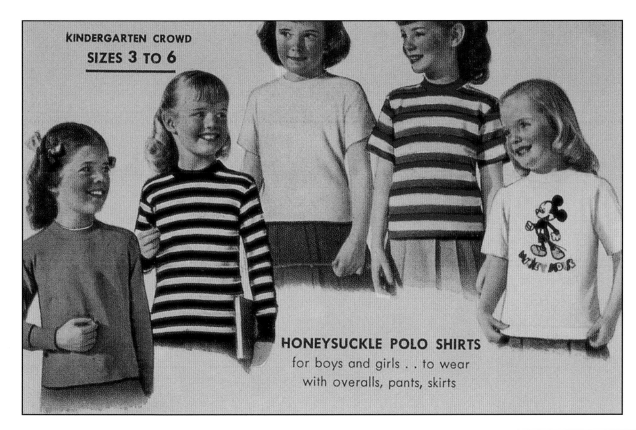

Honeysuckle polo shirts, for boys and girls to wear with overalls, pants, and skirts. Striped, solid, or character printed, great for under sweaters or jackets. $1-2. [$5-10] *Fall/winter 1948*

100% virgin wool jacquard patterns for girls and boys, each in pullover and cardigan. Knit patterns on back and front. $2-3. [$5-10] *Fall/winter 1948*

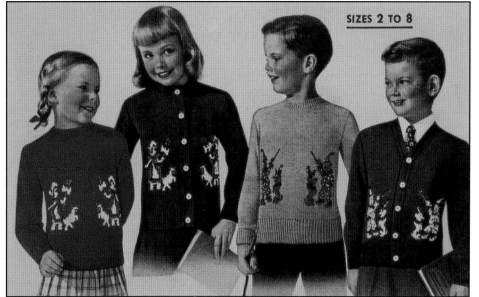

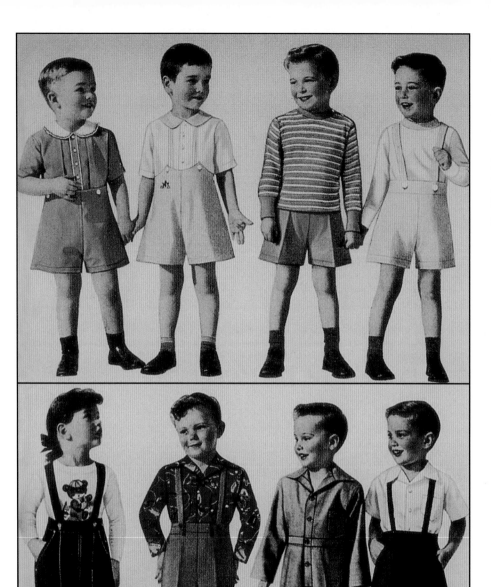

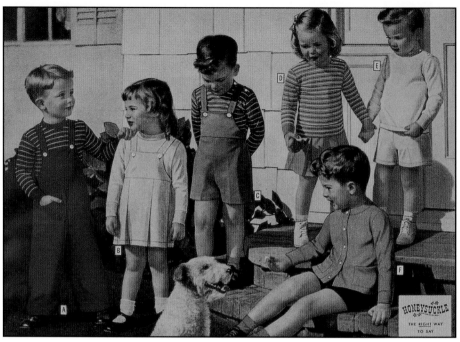

Knit cottons, mix or match separates for boys and girls…overalls, skirts, shorts, polo shirts, and sweaters, in the softest, finest styles. Pink, yellow, medium blue, red, or light blue. Anklet socks to match. $1-2. [$3-5] *Fall/winter 1948*

Toddlers' cotton poplin two-piece suits, button-on suspenders, denim dungarees, western "Rancho" style pants, Sanforized cotton twill or chambray playsuits, cotton gabardine, in sweet colors. $1-3. [$5-10] *Fall/winter 1948*

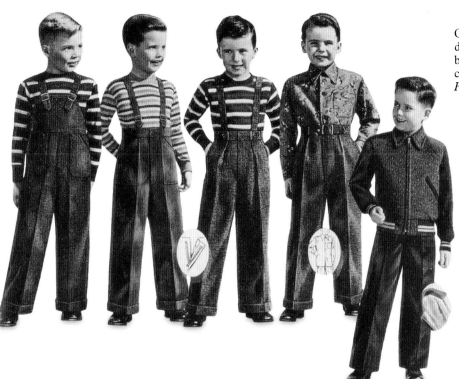

Corduroy, an idea fabric for active boys…tough as nails, won't show dirt, and stays nice looking. Suspender longies and bib pants, in dark brown or navy blue. Cotton knit polo shirts or cotton suede collared cowboy style shirts go great with these comfortable pants. $3-6. [$5-10]
Fall/winter 1948

Sanforized cotton fabrics specially selected for wear-resistance, well made for lively youngsters. Long sleeve styles for top-to-toe protection. Washfast blue chambray, Texas green washfast twill, washfast blue jean, or rugged hickory stripe. $1-2. [$5-10]
Fall/winter 1948

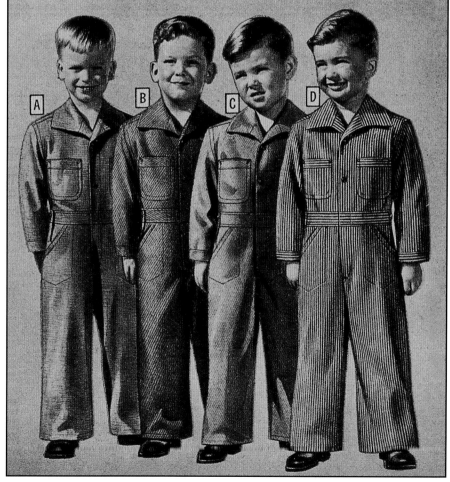

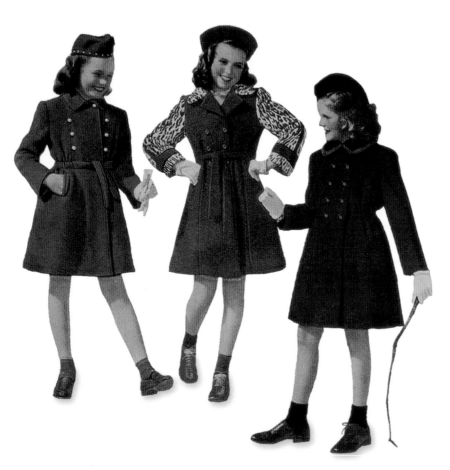

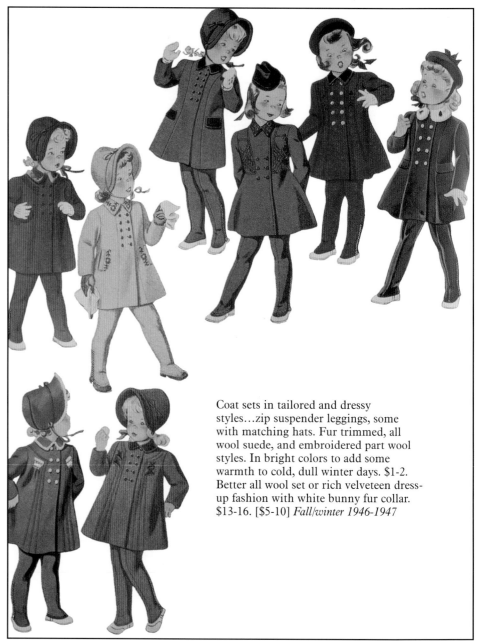

Better Honeylanes, new fall dressy styles. Pull through tie front Shetland-type wool, in royal or rosewine. Leopard print fabric sleeves and collar, and all wool domestic Shetland-type coating, in medium green or rosewine. Laskin lamb fur collar enriches a lovely all wool fleece style, in wine red or teal blue. Alpaca and wool blend coat, in medium brown. All virgin wool suede fleece jewel coat, in deep rose, cocoa brown, or bright green. $15-16. [$20-30] *Fall/winter 1946-1947*

Coat sets in tailored and dressy styles…zip suspender leggings, some with matching hats. Fur trimmed, all wool suede, and embroidered part wool styles. In bright colors to add some warmth to cold, dull winter days. $1-2. Better all wool set or rich velveteen dress-up fashion with white bunny fur collar. $13-16. [$5-10] *Fall/winter 1946-1947*

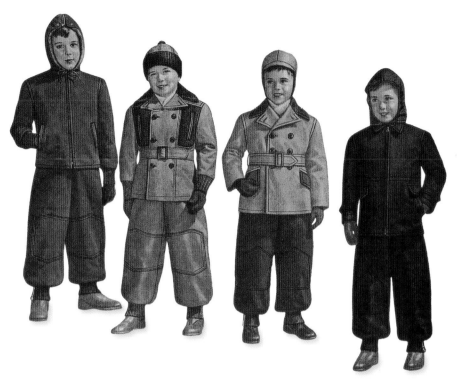

Get him ready for snow, rain, or sleet…the best Boyville Jr. outdoor suits, specially treated to repel moisture. Water-resistant heavy cotton twill, parka style, Zeland poplin and mountain cloth coats, with fluffy and warm sheepskin or deep pile lining. Bib ski pants have adjustable strings for a good fit and outside knee patches for more protection. $9-17. [$10-20] *Fall/winter 1946-1947*

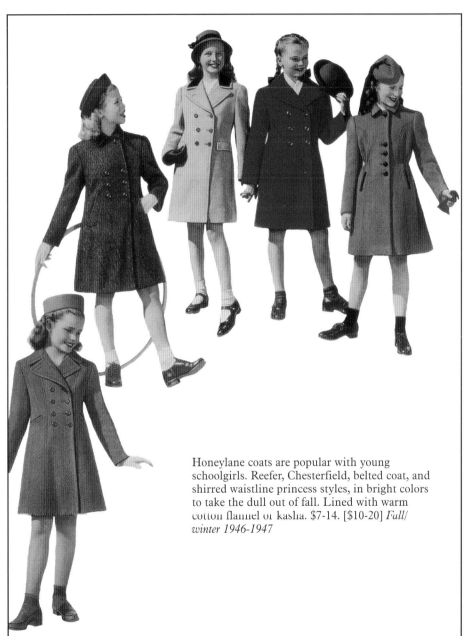

Honeylane coats are popular with young schoolgirls. Reefer, Chesterfield, belted coat, and shirred waistline princess styles, in bright colors to take the dull out of fall. Lined with warm cotton flannel or kasha. $7-14. [$10-20] *Fall/winter 1946-1947*

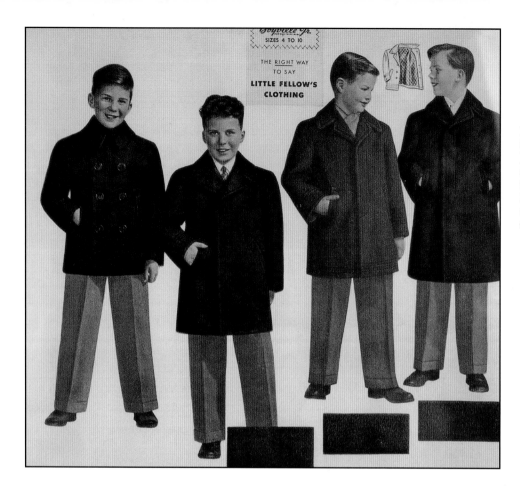

Dress-up styles that fellas like! Lined to give snug protection from Old Man Winter. All wool melton pea jacket, in navy blue. Warm Junior Fingertip coat, made of new wool, mohair, reprocessed wool, and rayon, in brown or teal. Junior Fingertip, best quality. Wool fleece face overcoat, quilted rayon body and sleeve linings in harmonizing colors. Canvas front and built-up shoulders for smart, comfortable fit, in beaver (dark brown) or teal. $7-13. [$15-20] *Fall/winter 1946-1947*

The cutest tricks that walk between the rain drops…from kindergarten to high school. Let Little Miss feel like a big girl with grown-up coats. Cotton gabardine fly front "boy" coat, smart and popular fashion, in tan, medium blue, or red. Rubberized cotton-hooded raincoat in colorful plaid. $2-5. [$5-10] *Spring/summer 1947*

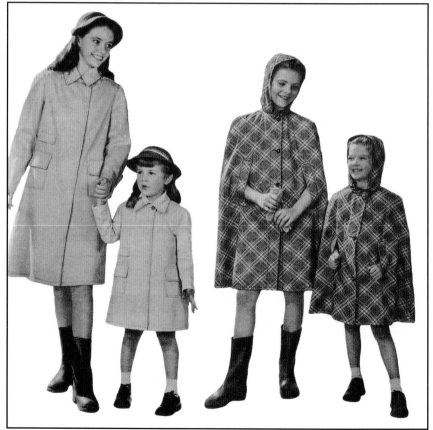

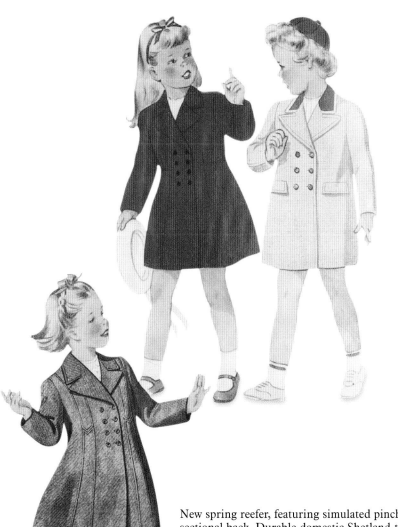

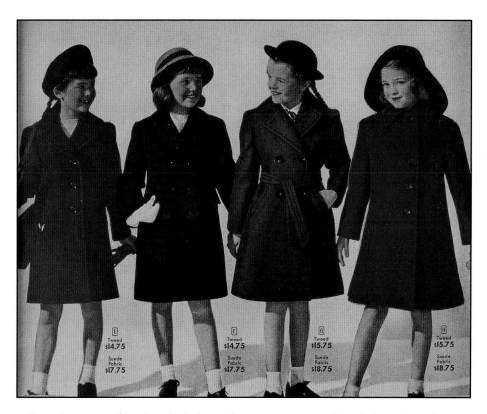

Honeylane coats of preshrunk virgin woolens, monotone tweed or virgin wool suede fabrics in clear, bright colors. Canvas lining, reversible collar. $15-19. [$15-20] *Fall/winter 1948*

New spring reefer, featuring simulated pinch drape and sectional back. Durable domestic Shetland-type all wool, in bright red or light blue. Double-breasted boy coat, 100% wool, all dressed-up with bright red contrasting collar and matching red buttons, light gray. $6-8. [$5-10] *Spring/summer 1947*

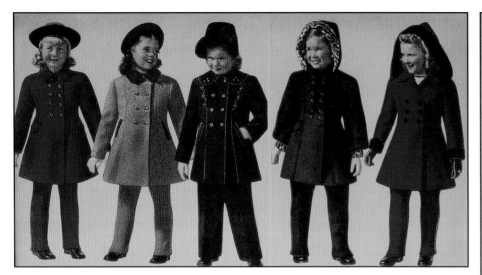

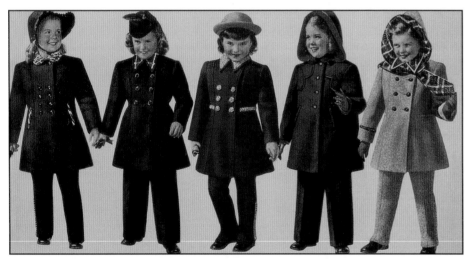

Honeysuckle coat and legging sets in warm, long-wearing all wool fabrics. Coats have rayon linings and warm cotton interlinings, leggings have adjustable buckle suspenders and are warmly lined with cotton kasha. Grown-up styles to make her feel big. $12-18. [$15-20] *Fall/winter 1948*

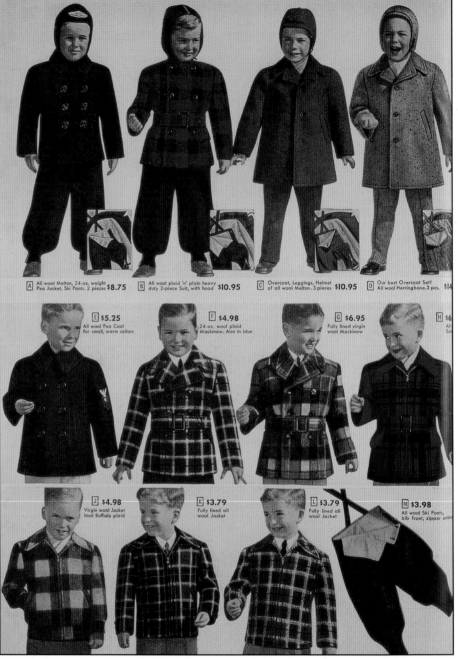

A All wool Melton, 24-oz. weight Pea Jacket, Ski Pants. 2 pieces **$8.75**   B All wool plaid 'n' plain heavy duty 2-piece Suit, with hood **$10.95**   C Overcoat, Leggings, Helmet of all wool Melton. 3 pieces **$10.95**   D Our best Overcoat Set! All wool Herringbone. 3 pcs. **$14**

E **$5.25** All wool Pea Coat for small, warm sailors   F **$4.98** 24-oz. wool plaid Mackinaw. Also in blue   G **$6.95** Fully lined virgin wool Mackinaw   H **$6** All Sur

J **$4.98** Virgin wool Jacket loud Buffalo plaid   K **$3.79** Fully lined all wool Jacket   L **$3.79** Fully lined all wool Jacket   M **$3.98** All wool Ski Pants, bib front, zipper ankle

Outdoor suits and overcoat sets by Boyville Jr. All wool melton pea jackets, all wool plaid 'n' heavy duty suit with hood, wool plaid, fully-lined Mackinaw, all wool surcoat, and virgin wool jacket with buffalo plaid and zipper front. Ski pants with bib front to match any of the coats. $5-15. [$10-15] *Fall/winter 1948*

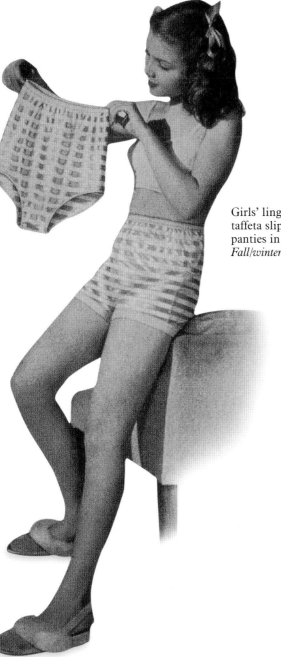

Girls' lingerie…rayon satin or rayon taffeta slips, in tearose. Knit rayon panties in cuff or brief styles. $1. [$1] *Fall/winter 1946-1947*

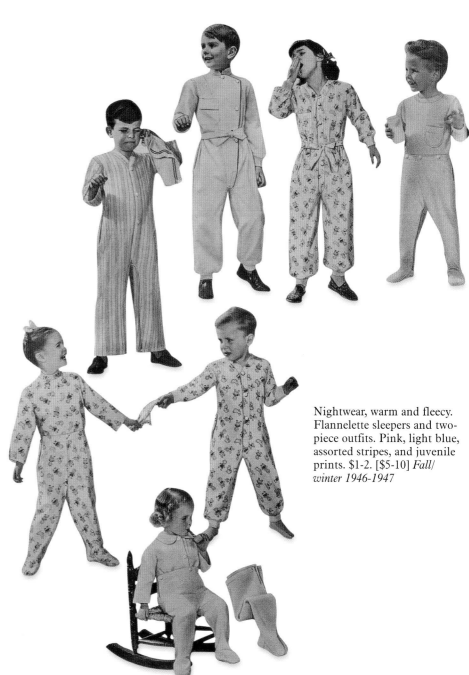

Nightwear, warm and fleecy. Flannelette sleepers and two-piece outfits. Pink, light blue, assorted stripes, and juvenile prints. $1-2. [$5-10] *Fall/winter 1946-1947*

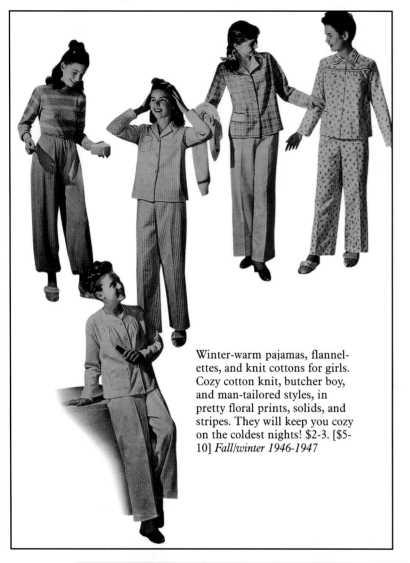

Winter-warm pajamas, flannel-ettes, and knit cottons for girls. Cozy cotton knit, butcher boy, and man-tailored styles, in pretty floral prints, solids, and stripes. They will keep you cozy on the coldest nights! $2-3. [$5-10] *Fall/winter 1946-1947*

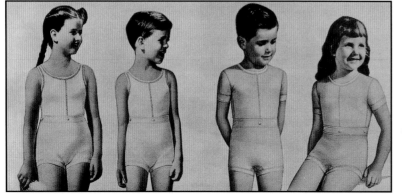

Style-right swim suits, a colorful parade of the gay, flattering fashions girls like for swimming or sunning. Printed rayon sharkskin in princess style or multicolor print. One-piece suit knit of rayon and cotton in velvet-like texture, with snowy daisy chain braid trim on neck and

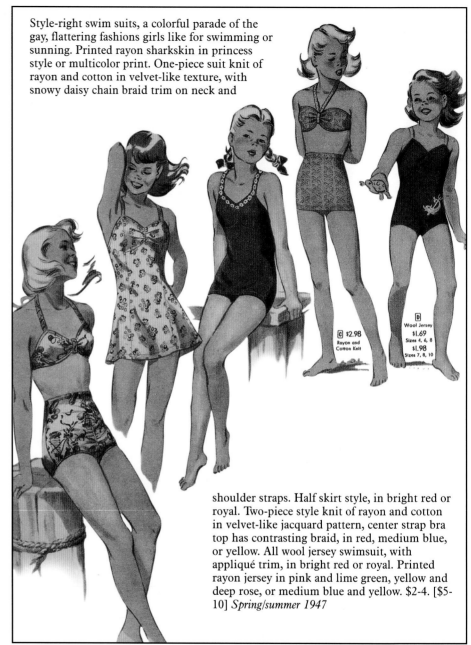

shoulder straps. Half skirt style, in bright red or royal. Two-piece style knit of rayon and cotton in velvet-like jacquard pattern, center strap bra top has contrasting braid, in red, medium blue, or yellow. All wool jersey swimsuit, with appliqué trim, in bright red or royal. Printed rayon jersey in pink and lime green, yellow and deep rose, or medium blue and yellow. $2-4. [$5-10] *Spring/summer 1947*

Honeysuckle knit underwear…vests stay tucked in, panties stay up! Lightweight cotton sleeveless vest and brief panties, or medium weight combed cotton short-sleeve vest and brief panties, in dainty tearose shade for girls and white for boys or girls. $1. [$1] *Spring/summer 1947*

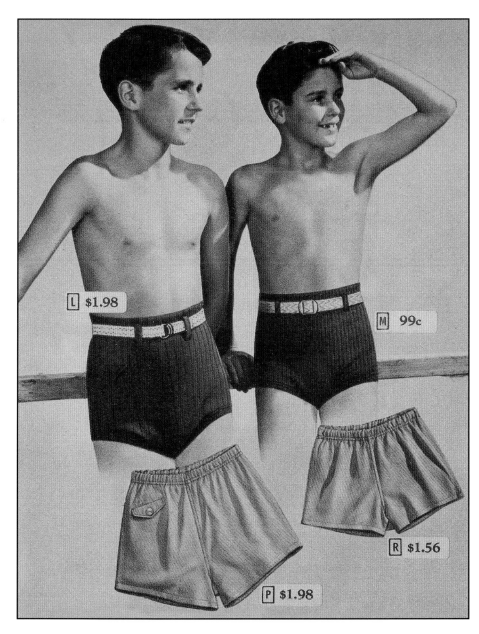

L $1.98

M 99c

R $1.56

P $1.98

Boyville swim trunks…they'll give him summers of wear. All wool or part wool close-fitting knitted style, or boxer model trunks with elastic drawstring waist, made of good cotton gabardine. In medium tan, maize (yellow), medium blue, or maroon. $1-2. [$3-5] *Spring/summer 1947*

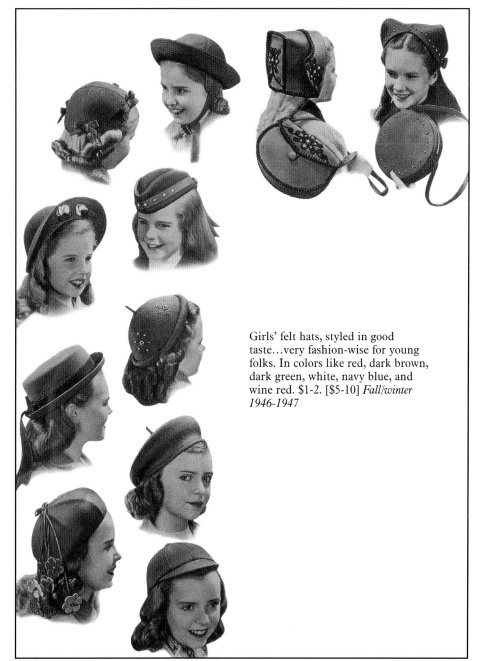

Girls' felt hats, styled in good taste…very fashion-wise for young folks. In colors like red, dark brown, dark green, white, navy blue, and wine red. $1-2. [$5-10] *Fall/winter 1946-1947*

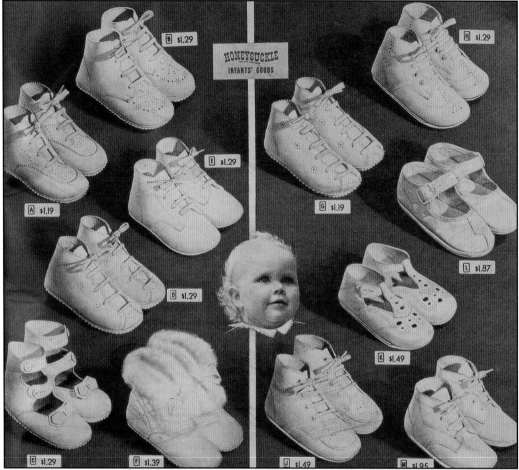

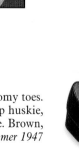

Babies' soft sole shoes, constructed for growing feet. Moc-type, roman sandal, slip-ons, blucher-style creepers, and fur-trimmed boots. White. $1-2. [$1-3] *Spring/summer 1947*

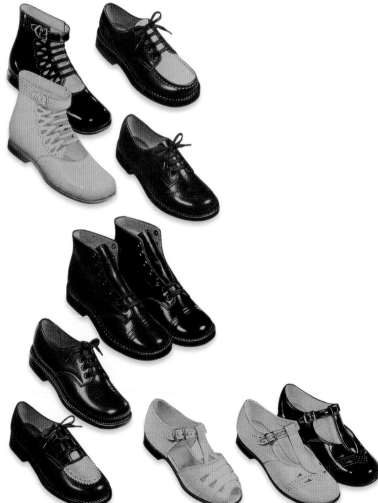

Biltwels for boys and girls…flexible soles, fine leathers, and roomy toes. Moc-type high shoe, playtime saddles, clean-cut oxford, shield tip huskie, sugar 'n' spice in patent leather T-strap sandal, and ghillie tie. Brown, white, or black leather. $2-5. [$5-10] *Spring/summer 1947*

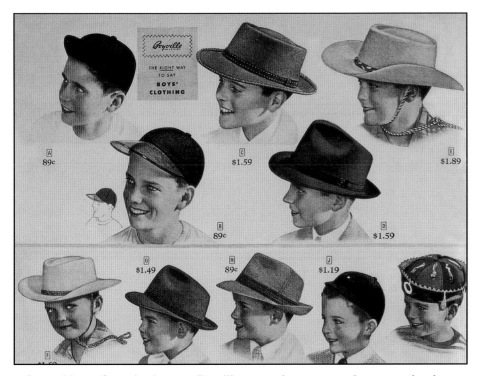

Spruce him up for spring in smart Boyville accessories…sports style caps, cowboy hats, and dress hats, for all occasions. $1-2. [$5-10] *Spring/summer 1947*

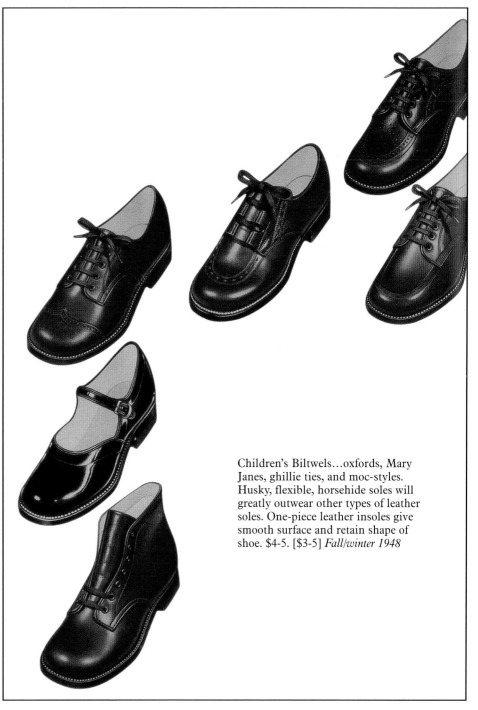

Children's Biltwels…oxfords, Mary Janes, ghillie ties, and moc-styles. Husky, flexible, horsehide soles will greatly outwear other types of leather soles. One-piece leather insoles give smooth surface and retain shape of shoe. $4-5. [$3-5] *Fall/winter 1948*

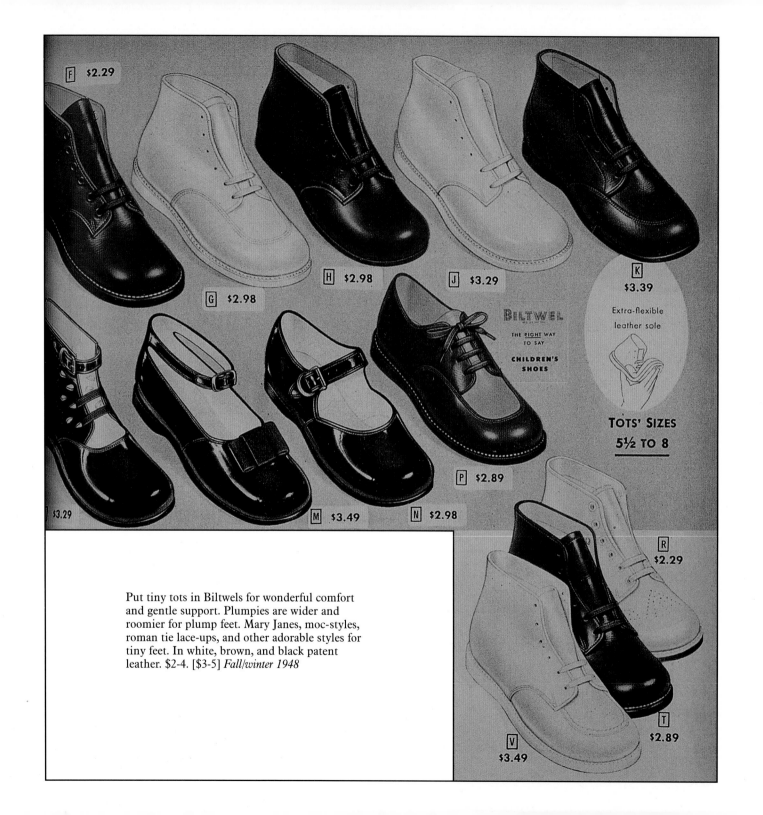

F $2.29

G $2.98

H $2.98

J $3.29

K $3.39
Extra-flexible leather sole

BILTWEL
THE RIGHT WAY TO SAY
CHILDREN'S SHOES

TOTS' SIZES 5½ TO 8

$3.29

M $3.49

N $2.98

P $2.89

R $2.29

T $2.89

V $3.49

Put tiny tots in Biltwels for wonderful comfort and gentle support. Plumpies are wider and roomier for plump feet. Mary Janes, moc-styles, roman tie lace-ups, and other adorable styles for tiny feet. In white, brown, and black patent leather. $2-4. [$3-5] *Fall/winter 1948*